Contents

Easy EMG

A Guide to Performing Nerve Conduction Studies and Electromyography

Edited by

Lyn Weiss MD

Chairman and Director of Residency Training;
Professor of Clinical Physical Medicine and Rehabilitation;
Director of Electrodiagnostic Services
Department of Physical Medicine and Rehabilitation
Nassau University Medical Center
East Meadow, NY, USA

Julie Silver MD

Assistant Professor
Department of Physical Medicine and Rehabilitation
Harvard Medical School
Boston, MA, USA

Jay Weiss MD

Medical Director
Long Island Physical Medicine and Rehabilitation
Levittown, NY, USA

Illustrator:

Dennis Dowling DO

Chairman and Professor
The Stanley Schiowitz Department of Osteopathic Manipulative Medicine
New York College Osteopathic Medicine
New York Insitute of Technology
Old Westbury, NY, USA

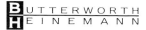

A Division of Elsevier Inc

Edinburgh London New York Oxford Philadelphia St Louis Sydney Toronto 2004

BUTTERWORTH-HEINEMANN
An imprint of Elsevier Inc

First published 2004

ISBN 0750674318

British Library Cataloguing in Publication Data
A catalogue record for this book is available from the British Library

Library of Congress Cataloging in Publication Data
A catalog record for this book is available from the Library of Congress

Notice
Medical knowledge is constantly changing. Standard safety precautions must be followed, but as new research and clinical experience broaden our knowledge, changes in treatment and drug therapy may become necessary or appropriate. Readers are advised to check the most current product information provided by the manufacturer of each drug to be administered to verify the recommended dose, the method and duration of administration, and contraindications. It is the responsibility of the practitioner, relying on experience and knowledge of the patient, to determine dosages and the best treatment for each individual patient. Neither the Publisher nor the editors/contributors assumes any liability for any injury and/or damage to persons or property arising from this publication.

The Publisher

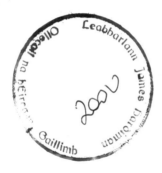

The publisher's policy is to use **paper manufactured from sustainable forests**

Printed in China

Contributors

Dennis Dowling DO
Chairman and Professor
The Stanley Schiowitz Department of
Osteopathic Manipulative Medicine
New York College of Osteopathic
Medicine
New York Institute of Technology
Old Westbury, NY, USA

Carlo Esteves MD DO
Fellow, Pain Medicine
Pacific Pain Treatment Center
San Francisco, CA, USA

Rebecca Fishman DO
Chief of Physical Medicine and
Rehabilitation
New York College of Osteopathic
Medicine
New York Institute of Technology
Old Westbury, NY, USA

Nancy Fung MD
Assistant Attending Physician
New York Weill Cornell Center
New York Presbyterian Hospital
New York, NY, USA

Walter Gaudino MD
Associate Professor of Clinical Physical
Medicine and Rehabilitation
Associate Chairman, Department of
Physical Medicine and Rehabilitation
Nassau University Medical Center
East Meadow, NY, USA

Kristin Gustafson DO
Chief Resident, Department of Physical
Medicine and Rehabilitation

Nassau University Medical Center
East Meadow, NY, USA

Victor Isaac MD
Resident, Department of Physical
Medicine and Rehabilitation
Nassau University Medical Center
East Meadow, NY, USA

Arthur Kalman DO
SHANDS at the University of Florida
Gainesville, FL, USA

David Khanan MD
Private Practice
Long Island, NY

Thomas Pobre MD
Assistant Professor of Clinical
Physical Medicine and
Rehabilitation
Director of Outpatient Physical
Medicine and Rehabilitation
Nassau University Medical Center
East Meadow, NY, USA

Chaim Shtock MD DO
Resident, Department of Physical
Medicine and Rehabilitation
Nassau University Medical Center
East Meadow, NY, USA

Julie K Silver MD
Assistant Professor
Department of Physical Medicine and
Rehabilitation
Harvard Medical School
Boston, MA, USA

Limeng Wang MD
Resident, Department of Physical
Medicine and Rehabilitation
Nassau University Medical Center
East Meadow, NY, USA

Lyn Weiss MD
Chairman and Director of Residency
Training;
Professor of Clinical Physical Medicine
and Rehabilitation;
Director of Electrodiagnostic Services
Department of Physical Medicine and
Rehabilitation
Nassau University Medical Center
East Meadow, NY, USA

Jay Weiss MD
Medical Director
Long Island Physical Medicine and
Rehabilitation
Levittown, NY, USA

Jie Zhu MD
Interventional Pain Fellow
Comprehensive Pain Center
Allentown, PA, USA

Preface

This book is the brainchild of a Physical Medicine and Rehabilitation resident who, early in her training, was frustrated by the lack of understandable electrodiagnostic medicine textbooks. There are many excellent texts that describe the theory and practice of electrodiagnostic medicine. However, this book is intended to be used by physicians who are just starting their training. This is not meant to be a comprehensive text. It is meant, rather, to serve as a bridge to more in-depth textbooks.

The first three chapters are introductory in nature. They briefly review what EMG testing is and why we do it. Chapter 4 assesses nerve conduction studies. The needle portion of the examination is discussed in Chapter 5. Chapter 6 reviews the effect of injury on peripheral nerves. Suggestions on how to plan out the examination are reviewed in Chapter 7. Chapter 8 examines some of the pitfalls that may befall both the novice and the more experienced electromyographer.

Chapters 9 through 20 review some of the commonly encountered clinical entities that the beginning electromyographer might encounter. Chapter 21 gives suggestions on how to write a complete electrodiagnostic report. Chapter 22 details the commonly accepted normal values for electrodiagnostic labs. It should be stressed however, that each lab should develop its own set of normals based on its own particular patient population and electrodiagnostic equipment. Reimbursement issues are discussed in Chapter 23.

It should be noted that this does not represent the complete spectrum of electrodiagnostic testing. Since this book is specifically targeted at novices in the field, some of the more complex testing, including somatosensory evoked potentials, blink reflex, and single fiber EMG, is not discussed.

Although this text does review a great deal of technical information, the most important lesson one can learn, which is stressed repeatedly throughout the text, is that the electrodiagnostic test is an extension of the history and physical examination. We are, first and foremost, physicians, with an obligation to provide our patients with compassionate and quality care.

Lyn Weiss, MD

Acknowledgments

Thank you, Sheila Slezak for your dedication, intelligence and good nature. You are an editor, investigator and computer whiz, all rolled into one super-secretary.

Thank you, Lisa Krivickas, MD, for your assistance in editing this book.

Jie Zhu deserves recognition for his work on the many tables in this text.

Special appreciation to Rebecca Fishman, DO, who was the impetus for this book. You have intellectual curiosity, the drive to get things accomplished and the personality to get people to cooperate.

Lyn Weiss, MD

1

What is an EMG?

Julie Silver

Electrodiagnostic studies seem very confusing at first. Remember this: the entire purpose of electrodiagnostic studies is to help you figure out whether there is a problem in the nervous system and if so, where the problem is occurring (Fig. 1.1). Easy to say, but we all recognize that the nervous system is a complicated part of our anatomy. Indeed, many medical students and residents find their initial exposure to these tests and the courses in which they are taught overwhelming. But the truth is that they are fairly straightforward and easy to understand.

If you don't believe this, think back to when you were a small child learning to read. At first all of the letters in the alphabet didn't make sense. Some had loops, some had straight lines, some had angled lines and some had all of these. But once you figured out all the letters, suddenly you could look at them anywhere and they made sense to you. Of course, you still couldn't read. That came later. But, even after you learned the alphabet, the higher-level task of reading (at some point not too long after you learned the alphabet) eventually became a breeze. So, too, will electrodiagnostic studies.

Think of the first half of this book as learning the alphabet. You will need to simply memorize some terms and try to understand when to use them and in what context they are meaningful – just like the alphabet letters. The second half of this book is the part where you learn to read or to put the things you have memorized to use in a logical way so that when electrodiagnostic studies are ordered, you can understand what information is being conveyed and how to perform the study. Keeping with the alphabet/reading example, more advanced electrodiagnostic textbooks will teach you the equivalent of grammar and higher level skills that are extremely important. However, you don't need to know all that at first. Go through every chapter in this book, and just like you learned the alphabet and then learned to read, you will become an expert at electrodiagnostic studies – only it will happen much faster this time!

The term *electrodiagnostic studies* really encompasses a lot of different tests. The most common tests done (and the ones that will be presented in this book) are nerve conduction studies (NCS) and electromyography (EMG). Often people refer to *both* NCS and EMG as *just* EMG because these two tests are nearly always done together. But, when you are talking with people who are familiar with electrodiagnostic testing, to avoid confusion it is best to speak of these components separately. The tests can provide different information, however, both tests assess the electrical functioning of nerves and/or muscles.

It is interesting to note that electrodiagnostic studies originated in the 19th century but have only been consistently used within the past 30–40 years. This is because the machines became more sophisticated with computerization, and at the same time, easier to use. Highly refined techniques enhanced diagnostic applications and encouraged people to use these tests.

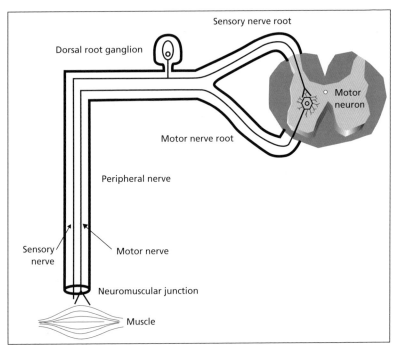

Figure 1.1 The goal of electrodiagnostic studies is to determine whether there is a problem along the peripheral nervous system pathway and if so, where the problem is. Examples of locations of possible lesions and associated diagnoses include:
Motor nerve cell body (anterior horn cell) – amyotrophic lateral sclerosis
Root – cervical or lumbar radiculopathy
Axon – toxic neuropathy
Myelin – Guillain–Barré syndrome
Neuromuscular junction – myasthenia gravis
Muscle – muscular dystrophy

One of the things that will make it much easier for you to learn both EMG and NCS is to understand that *they are really an extension of the neurological and musculoskeletal examination*. The more you know about the basic anatomy of the nerves and muscles, the easier it will be to learn about electrodiagnostic studies. If you are just beginning to learn about what nerves supply what muscles and such, this will be a slightly more complicated subject, but still very manageable. Just keep reading.

Table 1.1 is a summary of the process of performing electrodiagnostic studies. The rest of this chapter is devoted to explaining the two basic tests: EMG and NCS. Some of this you will simply need to memorize, but hopefully as you read, it will start to make sense.

 Nerve Conduction Studies

NCS are done by placing electrodes on the skin and stimulating the nerves through electrical impulses (Fig. 1.2). To study motor nerves, electrodes are placed over a muscle

Table 1.1 The electrodiagnostic process

1. Evaluate the patient by doing a history and physical examination with the goal of developing a differential diagnoses list.
2. Select the appropriate electrodiagnostic tests you want to perform in order to rule in or out diagnoses on your list.
3. Explain to the patient what the test will feel like and why it is being done.
4. Perform the study in a technically competent fashion, usually starting with the nerve conduction studies and then proceeding with the EMG.
5. Interpret the results in order to arrive at the correct diagnosis or to narrow your list of differential diagnoses.
6. Communicate the test results to the referring physician in a timely and meaningful manner.

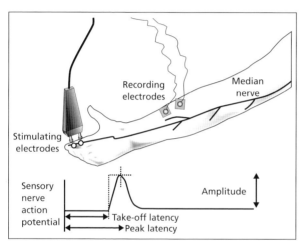

Figure 1.2 This is the basic set-up for a sensory nerve conduction study. The machine gives a tracing of the sensory nerve action potential (SNAP). The amplitude and latency can easily be measured. (Adapted from Misulis K. Essentials of Clinical Neurophysiology. London: Butterworth-Heinemann; 1997).

that receives its innervation from the nerve you want to test (stimulate). The electrical response of the muscle is then recorded and you can determine both how fast and how well the nerve responded. This is very valuable information and can help you to determine whether the patient's condition is stemming from a problem with the nerve or the muscle.

NCS are broken down into two categories: *motor* and *sensory* nerve conduction testing. The autonomic nervous system can be tested, but rarely has clinical applications and is beyond the scope of this text. NCS can be performed on any *accessible* nerve including peripheral nerves and cranial nerves. The basic findings are generally two-fold: 1. how fast is the impulse traveling? (e.g., how well is the electrical impulse conducting?); and, 2. what does the electrical representation of the nerve stimulation (action potential morphology) look like on the screen? (e.g., does there appear to be a problem with the shape or height that might suggest an injury to some portion of the nerve such as the axons or the myelin?).

Table 1.2 Nerve conduction study terms

Action potential – this is the waveform you see on the screen (in order to give more details about what you are describing, more specific terms may include compound nerve action potential, compound motor action potential, sensory nerve action potential, etc.)
Latency – time interval between the onset of a stimulus and the onset of a response (can also be referred to as a motor latency or a sensory latency).
Amplitude – the maximal height of the action potential.
Conduction velocity – how fast the fastest part of the impulse travels (can also be referred to as a motor conduction velocity or a sensory conduction velocity).
F-wave – a compound muscle action potential evoked by antidromically stimulating a motor nerve from a muscle using maximal electrical stimulus. It represents the time required for a stimulus to travel antidromically toward the spinal cord and return orthodromically to the muscle along a very small percentage of the fibers.
H-reflex – a compound muscle action potential evoked by orthodromically stimulating sensory fibers, synapsing at the spinal level and returning orthodromically via motor fibers. The response is thought to be due to a monosynaptic spinal reflex (Hoffmann reflex) found in normal adults in the gastrocnemius-soleus and flexor carpi radialis muscles.
Orthodromic – when the electrical impulse travels in the same direction as normal physiologic conduction (e.g., when a motor nerve electrical impulse is transmitted toward the muscle and away from the spine or a sensory impulse travels toward the spine).
Antidromic – when the electrical impulse travels in the opposite direction of normal physiologic conduction (e.g., conduction of a motor nerve electrical impulse away from the muscle and toward the spine).

The terms you need to memorize in NCS are listed in Table 1.2. EMG terms are listed and explained in Chapter 5 (Electromyography).

 ## Electromyography

EMG is the process by which an examiner puts a needle into a particular muscle and studies the electrical activity of that muscle. This electrical activity comes from the muscle itself – no shocks are used to stimulate the muscle. The EMG also differs from the NCS because it does not involve actually testing nerves. However, you do get information indirectly about the nerves by testing the muscles (remember that all muscles are supplied by nerves, so if you can identify which muscles are affected by a disease process then you simultaneously obtain information about the nerves that supply those muscles).

So, the EMG is different from NCS in the following ways:

1. You use a needle and put it into the muscle rather than electrodes that are placed on the skin.
2. You don't use any electrical shocks in EMG; rather you are looking at the *intrinsic* electrical activity of the muscle.
3. You get *direct* information about the muscles in EMG and *indirect* information about the nerves that supply the muscles you test.

2

Why do Electrodiagnostic Studies?

Julie Silver

Electrodiagnostic testing is an important method for physicians to distinguish between many nerve and muscle disorders. One of the ways to think of EMG and NCS is to consider them pieces of a puzzle. The puzzle may be complicated with many pieces or fairly straightforward with few pieces needed to solve it. In order to understand what you are seeing, whether it is a real puzzle or a figurative medical puzzle, the more pieces you can put into place, the clearer the picture becomes. In medicine, the other puzzle pieces are the history, physical examination, laboratory tests, imaging studies, etc.

One of the things that is important to remember is that electrodiagnostic studies represent a *physiologic* piece of the diagnostic puzzle. For example, unlike an MRI or an x-ray, which are simply sophisticated photographs, the EMG and NCS provide information in real time about what is occurring physiologically with respect to the nerve and the muscle. This is not to say that imaging studies are not useful, but rather to explain that these tests complement each other and each has a role in helping to establish the correct diagnosis in neuromuscular disorders.

The take-home message is this: Electrodiagnostic studies are sometimes essential in establishing a particular diagnosis and are sometimes not useful at all. As a clinician, it is important to understand when to recommend these studies just as it is important to know when to order an imaging study. The more you learn about EMG and NCS, the more familiar you will become with their diagnostic usefulness.

In a practical sense, you can consider electrodiagnostic testing in any of the following circumstances:

1. A patient is complaining of numbness.
2. A patient is complaining of tingling (paresthesias).
3. A patient has pain.
4. A patient has weakness.
5. A patient has a limp.
6. A patient has muscle atrophy.
7. A patient has depressed deep tendon reflexes.
8. A patient has fatigue.

Of course, it would be ridiculous to rely solely on any one of these signs or symptoms when recommending NCS/EMG. For example, a young woman comes in complaining of arm pain. The differential diagnosis should immediately include trauma as a source of the pain. Upon questioning you learn that in fact she fell and on physical examination you note a large abrasion that explains her pain. To even consider electrodiagnostic studies in this situation is absurd. The point here is that a list of signs and symptoms does not lead you to automatically order electrodiagnostic studies. Rather, these tests can be thought of as an *extension of the history and physical examination* when someone presents with any one or more of the signs or symptoms listed that cannot be explained by the history and physical examination alone.

Clearly electrodiagnostic studies are useful to establish the correct diagnosis, but they are also useful to determine whether someone should have surgery and are often preferred over imaging studies when certain types of surgery are a consideration. They are also done for prognostic reasons to follow the course of recovery (or deterioration) from an injury.

In summary, electrodiagnostic studies are used to:

1. Establish the correct diagnosis.
2. Localize the lesion.
3. Determine treatment even if the diagnosis is already known.
4. Provide information about the prognosis.
   Consider the following examples:

Example 1

A man comes in with hand pain, paresthesias and numbness that are most prominent in the index and long fingers. Upon questioning he also reveals he has neck pain. The physical examination is inconclusive. The differential diagnosis includes carpal tunnel syndrome (median nerve compression at the wrist) and cervical radiculopathy. An EMG and NCS are the studies of choice to establish the correct diagnosis.

Example 2

Another man comes in with the same symptoms but he doesn't have neck pain. In the past he was diagnosed with carpal tunnel syndrome and underwent an injection with local corticosteroid into the carpal tunnel that completely alleviated his symptoms for a few months (a good response to a corticosteroid injection in the carpal tunnel is both therapeutic and *diagnostic* for carpal tunnel syndrome). Now, however, his symptoms are back with a vengeance. In this case of carpal tunnel syndrome, electrodiagnostic studies can be recommended in order to determine the severity of his condition and to help decide whether conservative management or surgery is the most appropriate course of treatment.

Example 3

A third man comes in who had carpal tunnel surgery 3 months ago. His symptoms are much better, but he is still quite weak. Prior to his surgery he had an EMG and NCS that demonstrated a very severe injury to the median nerve. Now, he is a candidate for repeat electrodiagnostic studies to provide information about the prognosis. The new study can be compared to the old study, and information extrapolated about the current status of the median nerve and predicted future improvement.

The Skilled and Compassionate Electrodiagnostician

Many patients are afraid to have electrodiagnostic studies. They may have heard that these tests are extremely painful or they may have a genuine needle phobia. In order to get the information you need from these tests, it is important for you to be both technically skilled and able to put the patient at ease. The following suggestions will help to lessen the patient's anxiety:

1. Avoid keeping the patient waiting, as that will only increase his or her anxiety.
2. Before you start, explain to the patient what you are going to do. Be sure the patient understands that the electrical stimulation occurs *only* with the NCS and *not* with EMG.
3. Explain that these tests will be useful in determining the diagnosis.
4. Reassure the patient that you will stop the test at any point if they request you to do so. Be sure to honor the request should it occur.
5. Start with the area of greatest interest – especially if you suspect that the patient won't tolerate the entire study.
6. Although not typically used, analgesic or sedating medication can be given.
7. During the test, distract the patient with conversation. It is usually easy to distract someone by asking them questions about what they like to do, where they like to go, etc. Some electromyographers play music of the patient's choosing during the test.
8. In most instances, it is best not to show patients the needle as many people associate more pain with a long needle rather than with a larger diameter (the EMG needle is long and thin, so it really doesn't hurt as much as a larger diameter needle). In addition, most patients feel more comfortable with the term 'electrical stimulation' rather than 'electrical shock', which conjures up images of torture.
9. Assure the patient that you will minimize the length of the exam, doing only what is absolutely necessary to obtain the required information.
10. Keep the room warm. This serves two purposes. First of all, the patient is generally dressed in a gown and therefore is prone to being cold. Keeping the room warm will make him or her more comfortable. In addition, the results of your electrodiagnostic test may be affected if the patient's extremity is cool (see Chapter 8, Pitfalls).

Special Precautions

There are a number of clinical situations that deserve special mention. These are cases where electrodiagnostic studies can be safely done, as long as the physician takes measures to ensure the safety of the patient (and himself/herself) and the accuracy of the test.

Morbid Obesity

In patients who are very overweight, it may be difficult (or impossible) to localize specific muscles. Care must be taken to ensure that the needle is indeed placed in the appropriate muscle. Extra-long needles may be used.

Thin Individuals

In very thin patients, it is important not to insert the needle too far as it can injure other tissues (e.g., a needle placed in the thoracic paraspinals may penetrate the lungs and cause a pneumothorax).

Bleeding Disorders

Individuals with known bleeding disorders or who are on anticoagulation therapy should be assessed on an individual basis and the risks/benefits of the test evaluated. It may be helpful to have recent laboratory testing for coagulation parameters. Therapeutic levels of anticoagulation are not a contraindication to EMG.

Blood Precautions

It is imperative to always practice safe needle-stick procedures to protect yourself and the patient from injury. These include always wearing gloves for the needle portion of the test, using a sterile disposable needle for the EMG, using a one-handed technique if needed for needle recapping and immediately disposing of all sharps in an appropriate container.

Contraindications

Strict contraindications to electrodiagnostic testing are relatively few. Obviously anyone who has a severe bleeding disorder or whose anticoagulation therapy is out of control should not undergo an EMG. NES are contraindicated in those with automatic implanted cardiac defibrillators. A patient with a cardiac pacemaker should not receive direct electrical stimulation over the pacemaker. Someone with an active skin/soft tissue infection (e.g., cellulitis) should not have an EMG anywhere near the infection. There is controversy over whether someone who has had an axillary node dissection after a mastectomy should undergo any needle punctures in the affected extremity. The clinician should consider this a relative contraindication and weigh the risks/benefits of the study.

Complications

Complications from electrodiagnostic studies are extremely rare when performed by a skilled clinician. Complications may include infection, bleeding and accidental penetration of the needle into something other than the intended muscle (e.g., lung, nerves, etc.).

Controversy

As with nearly every test in medicine, there is controversy about when to do electrodiagnostic studies. There is no doubt that EMG and NCS provide valuable information and in many instances are worthwhile tests to pursue. However, they must be judiciously performed – as is the case with all medical testing. Of course, there would not be any controversy if these studies were painless and free. But this is not the case. They do cause some patient discomfort (although this can be minimized with a skilled and compassionate approach) and they are relatively expensive tests to perform. So, it is important every time you consider performing electrodiagnostic studies to assess whether the test is necessary, whether it will help you to determine the diagnosis, treatment or prognosis of a patient's condition, and whether there is another test that might be less intrusive and/or more cost effective that will provide the same information. It is important to always remember to *first do no harm.*

3
About the Machine

Julie Silver

The Basic Machine

Modern electrodiagnostic equipment consists of a computer and the associated hardware and software (Fig. 3.1). The hardware is fairly standard and typically includes a visual monitor, keyboard and hard and floppy disk drives. Some systems have additional hardware for storage and other purposes. The software varies in the same manner that all software varies – ease of use, ability to perform specific functions, etc. However, all basic electrodiagnostic software allows the clinician to:

- perform both EMG and NCS
- collect data
- help to analyze the results (through automatic calculations that are usually pre-programmed)
- store the information.

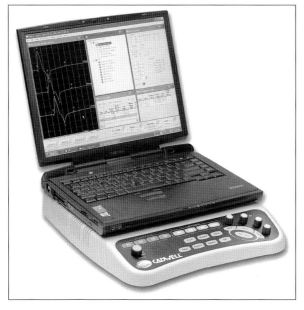

Figure 3.1 Picture of EMG machine (courtesy of Cadwell Laboratories).

Data entry is done using a keyboard and/or a mouse. When you are performing NCS, the information you need is displayed on a screen. During EMG studies, you will have the same visual screen information but also there will be audio (noises) that you will hear. Both the visual and the audio data are critical to properly interpreting EMG findings.

Recording Electrodes

It is important to understand electrode terms used in electrodiagnostic studies. Table 3.1 lists the common terms and in which studies they are used.

Surface Electrodes

Surface electrodes are used for routine NCS. The electrodes are typically either *ring* or *disk* electrodes (Fig. 3.2). They are also either *disposable* or *non-disposable*. The non-disposable electrodes are made of stainless steel, silver or – rarely – gold that is soldered to multistrand conducting wires. These electrodes stick to the skin by using adhesive tape and can be reused. They should be cleaned between patients. It is necessary to use conducting gel with *non-disposable* electrodes in order to reduce impedance and prevent artifact (due to irregularities in the skin and the presence of hair follicles). *Disposable* electrodes have a sticky underside that allows them to adhere to the skin without the need for tape or gel.

Three surface electrodes are used in NCS: active and reference recording electrodes and a ground electrode. In EMG studies, surface electrodes are used for the ground and sometimes as a reference-recording electrode.

Needle Electrodes

Needle electrodes are generally reserved for EMG, but are occasionally used in NCS. Today *nearly all needle electrodes are disposable and are used only on one patient.* Needle electrodes are classified as monopolar, bipolar or concentric. Monopolar needles are typically less expensive, less painful (due to a narrower diameter, and a teflon coating on the shaft of the needle) and less electrically stable than bipolar or concentric needle electrodes. With a monopolar needle, you need a separate surface reference electrode whereas with a concentric needle, the reference is the barrel of the needle and you do not need a separate surface reference electrode. See Chapter 5 (Electromyography) for further description of the needles.

Table 3.1 Electrodes used in NCS and EMG

NCS   Active (surface electrode – this is also referred to as the pickup electrode)   Reference (surface electrode)   Ground (surface electrode)
EMG   Active (needle electrode)   Reference (surface electrode)*   Ground (surface electrode)
*A separate reference is used in EMG studies only if you are using a monopolar needle. Concentric needles have a reference built into the needle, so there is no need for a separate reference.

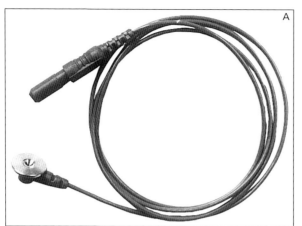

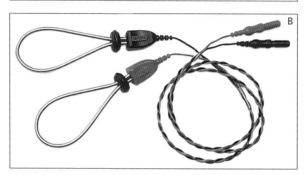

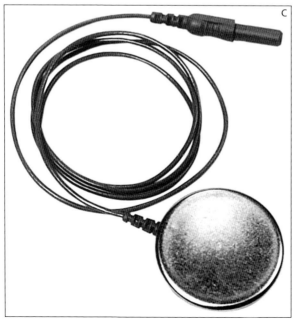

Figure 3.2 A, Disk electrade; B, ring electrode; C, ground electrode. (courtesy of Cadwell Laboratories).

Amplifiers

Amplifiers are a very complicated part of the electrodiagnostic machinery, but the concept is fairly simple. *Amplifiers magnify the signal so that it can be displayed* (Fig. 3.3). Integrated circuits or chips perform most amplification. *Preamplifiers* attenuate the biological signal before it ever gets to the amplifier in order to: 1. make sure that the filters have sufficient signal voltage to deal with, and 2. insure that the level of signal voltage is much higher than that of system noise.[1] The signal travels first to the pre-amplifier, then to the filters, and then to the amplifier. The *differential* amplifier is used extensively in electrodiagnostic studies, because it has the advantage of *common mode rejection*. What this means is that unwanted signals, rather than being amplified to the same degree as the biological signals that you are trying to study, are rejected. The most common unwanted signal in the clinic is 60-Hz activity, which is caused by line voltage passing through electrical circuits.

The differential amplifier takes the electrical impulses from the active electrode and amplifies them. It then takes the impulses from the reference electrode, inverts them, and amplifies them. It then combines these two potentials. In this way, any common noise to both electrodes (extraneous electrical activity, distant myogenic noise, and EKG artifacts) would be eliminated. Differences between the two electrodes, however, would be amplified. This is the desired signal. Any common factors such as extraneous noise would be rejected leading to the term *common mode rejection*. The common mode rejection ratio is a measure of how well an amplifier eliminates this type of common noise.

Filters

Filters are used to *faithfully reproduce the signal you want while trying to exclude both high and low frequency electrical noise.*[2] Every signal in both NCS and EMG passes through both a low frequency and a high frequency filter before being displayed. *Low frequency* filters are called *high pass* because they let high frequency signals pass

Figure 3.3
Preamplifier
(courtesy of
Cadwell
Laboratories).

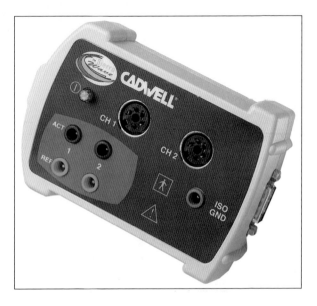

through. The range at which there is a cut-off of low frequency signals depends on how you set the filter. Similarly, *high frequency* filters are called *low pass* because they let low frequency signals through. It is important to understand that there is always a trade-off when you use filters. The signal you want will be altered to some degree. For example, as the low frequency filter is reduced, more low frequency signals pass through and the duration of the recorded potential will be slightly longer. Likewise, if the high frequency filter is decreased, more high frequency signals are excluded and the latency of the recorded potential may be delayed. Table 3.2 summarizes the role of filters and gives the usual settings in NCS and EMG.

 ## Display System

Display systems for electrodiagnostic studies are either via a video screen (computer screen) or paper. New display systems (e.g., liquid crystal, digital, etc.) are being developed, but the standard display is the *cathode ray tube* (CRT). The CRT uses a controlled electron beam (called the cathode ray) to excite phosphors on the screen that presents as a visual display. There are two settings on the display system with which you must be acquainted – the *sweep speed* and *sensitivity* (also sometimes called the *gain)*. The primary purpose of adjusting the sweep speed and sensitivity is so that you can optimally see the signal displayed on the screen. The *horizontal* axis is the *sweep speed* and is shown in milliseconds (ms) (Fig. 3.4). The *vertical* axis is the *sensitivity* and this represents response amplitude (millivolts in motor studies and microvolts in sensory studies) (Fig. 3.5). Suggested motor NCS settings are listed in Table 3.3. The initial settings for sensory NCS are listed in Table 3.4.

Table 3.2 Filters

Low frequency	High pass	Filters out low frequency signals that if present, cause a wandering baseline
High frequency	Low pass	Filters out high frequency signals that if present, can obscure signals such as SNAPs or fibrillation potentials and can cause a 'noisy' baseline especially on sensory studies

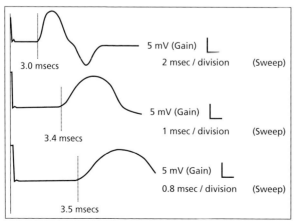

Figure 3.4 Effects of latency with changes in sweep speed (adapted from Preston DC, Shapiro BE. Electromyography and Neuromuscular Disorders. London: Butterworth-Heinemann, 1998).

Figure 3.5 Effect of increasing the sensitivity (gain) of a CMAP (adapted from Preston DC, Shapiro BE. Electromyography and Neuromuscular Disorders. London: Butterworth-Heinemann, 1998).

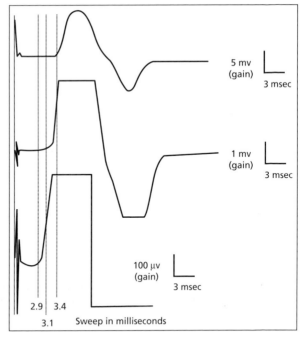

Table 3.3 Initial *motor* NCS settings*

Sweep speed	2–3 ms/div
Sensitivity (gain)	5000 microvolts/division (this means the same as 5 millivolts, 5mV or 5K microvolts)
Low frequency filter	10 Hz
High frequency filter	10 kHz
*Adapted from Misulis K. Essentials of Clinical Neurophysiology. London: Butterworth-Heinemann; 1997)	

Table 3.4 Initial *sensory* NCS settings*

Sweep speed	1 2 ms/div – generally 10 divisions are present in a horizontal screen
Sensitivity (gain)	20 microvolts/division
Low frequency filter	2–10 Hz
High frequency filter	2 kHz
*Adapted from Misulis K. Essentials of Clinical Neurophysiology. London: Butterworth-Heinemann; 1997)	

Artifacts and Technical Factors

Physiologic Factors (patient-related)

Stimulus Artifact

Stimulus artifact is an electrically recorded response that is elicited directly from the stimulator. It occurs in all NCS, however, it only becomes a problem when the trailing

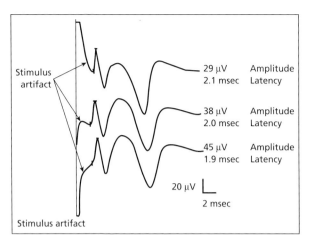

Figure 3.6 Large stimulus artifact may falsely decrease the amplitude and increase the latency (adapted from Preston DC, Shapiro BE. Electromyography and Neuromuscular Disorders. London: Butterworth-Heinemann, 1998).

edge of the recorded artifact overlaps with the potential being recorded (Fig. 3.6). Making sure the ground is between the recording and stimulating electrodes can minimize stimulus artifact.

Filters

Filters were discussed earlier in this chapter, but they are mentioned here because they can significantly contribute to the quality of your study. It is important to remember that the role of filters is to *faithfully reproduce the signal you want while trying to exclude both high and low frequency electrical noise.*

Electrode Placement

There are many issues that occur when electrodes are improperly placed. This discussion will be detailed throughout the rest of the book. Suffice it to say here that proper electrode placement is a critical part of performing accurate electrodiagnostic studies.

Stimulation

An important concept in NCS is to understand *supramaximal stimulation*. The bottom line is this: all measurements made in NCS are done with the assumption that the *strength* of the stimulus is high enough to depolarize every axon in the nerve. This is achieved by gradually increasing the stimulus strength until you reach the point where the amplitude of the waveform is no longer increasing. That is the point of supramaximal stimulation. If supramaximal stimulation is not achieved at a distal site, then you might mistakenly interpret this recording as signifying axonal loss due to the low amplitude. At a proximal site, this might appear to be *conduction block* (failure of an action potential to be conducted past a particular point whereas conduction is possible below the point of the block). In both instances, anomalous innervation or nerve injury may be wrongly suspected.

Of course, the old adage, too much of a good thing is not good, applies to many things in life. When it comes to stimulation in NCS, too much stimulation may cause co-stimulation of adjacent nerves or may stimulate nerves farther from the site. So, the goal is to reach supramaximal stimulation without applying so much stimulation that adjacent nerves are also stimulated.

Measurements

The machine will do most of your calculations for you. But you still need to measure the distance between stimulations and between the stimulation and the recording electrode of a patient's limb when you are determining the conduction velocity. It is imperative that the measurement is done accurately. Other than a simple oversight of not correctly recording the distance with your tape measure, the main problem that can occur is if the patient's limb is moved in different positions, which changes the distance you are measuring. This commonly occurs in ulnar nerve studies when the elbow is straight and then becomes flexed. Therefore, during an ulnar nerve study, it is best to keep the elbow flexed and in the same position for the duration of that particular study. Skin measurements are a major source of error in electrodiagnostic studies. This can be minimized by increasing the distance of the nerve segment being studied (i.e., the shorter the distance, the greater the effect of a measurement error). In general, when measuring distance, follow the course of the nerve, rather than measuring the shortest distance between the stimulating and recording electrodes.

Sweep Speed and Sensitivity

Both the sweep speed and sensitivity can affect your NCS results. As the sensitivity is increased, the onset latency will decrease. So, it is important to record all of your latency measurements using the same sensitivity and sweep speed.

REFERENCES

1. Misulis KE. Essentials of Clinical Neurophysiology. Newton, Massachusetts: Butterworth-Heinemann, 1997.
2. Preston DC, Shapiro, BE. Electromyography and Neuromuscular Disorders. Newton, Massachusetts: Butterworth-Heinemann, 1998.

4

Nerve Conduction Studies

Lyn Weiss, Jay Weiss, Thomas Pobre, Arthur Kalman

Nerve conduction studies (NCS) can be defined as *the recording of a peripheral neural impulse at some location distant from the site where a propagating action potential is induced in a peripheral nerve*. In other words, a nerve is stimulated at one or more sites along its course and the electrical response of the nerve is recorded.

Whether or not a nerve is injured can be evaluated by testing the ability of the nerve to conduct an electrical impulse. Nerve conduction studies allow us to accurately localize focal lesions or detect generalized disease processes along accessible portions of the peripheral nervous system. The reliability of a study is increased when the technical aspects of the study are standardized. This chapter will review why it can be helpful to utilize nerve conduction studies and how to perform them.

The nerve conduction studies most commonly performed are *compound muscle action potentials* (CMAPs) for motor nerves, *sensory nerve action potentials* (SNAPs) for sensory nerves, *compound nerve action potentials* (CNAPs) for mixed (sensory and motor) nerves and *late responses* (primarily F-waves and H-reflexes). For a discussion of F-waves and H-reflexes, see Chapter 12, Radiculopathy.

Physiology

When doing nerve conduction studies it is important to understand nerve physiology. After all, nerve studies are a physiological, not anatomic, test such as x-rays. In order to test nerve function we must understand how nerves conduct signals.

Nerves conduct impulses through a traveling wave of depolarization along their axon. The axon is the peripheral extension of the proximally located nerve cell body. The cell body is located in the spinal cord for motor nerves (anterior horn cell) and peripherally in the dorsal root ganglion for sensory nerves (Fig. 4.1). The surface membrane surrounding the axon is called axolemma, and contained within the axon is the axoplasm. At rest, the axon has an intracellular potential that is negative in relation to the extracellular potential. When an axon is conducting an impulse, voltage-dependent channels open and allow an influx of sodium (Na^+) ions. This influx of positive ions depolarizes the axon, changes the resting potential further down the axon, causing those channels to open and thus creates a wave of depolarization (Fig. 4.2).

While nerves have a physiological direction (*from* the spine in the case of motor nerves and *to* the spine in the case of sensory nerves), if a nerve is electrically stimulated anywhere along its course, waves of depolarization will travel in both directions from that point. Nerve conduction can be measured *orthodromically* (physiological direction of nerve conduction) or *antidromically* (opposite to the physiological direction). Motor and sensory nerve action potentials can be measured through skin electrodes if the nerve is

Figure 4.1 Cell body of sensory and motor nerves.

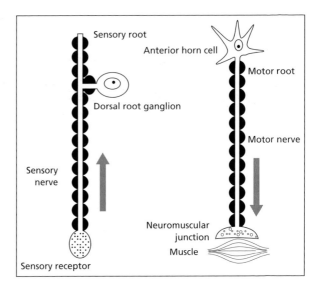

Figure 4.2 Wave of depolarization.

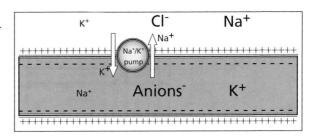

sufficiently superficial. It is more common (and technically easier) to measure motor nerves by picking up electrical activity from the muscle it innervates.

As a rule, nerve conduction study is done only on myelinated nerve fibers because unmyelinated fibers conduct extremely slowly, and do not contribute significantly to the CMAPs and SNAPs. A myelinated nerve fiber is composed of an axon and its surrounding myelin sheath (Fig. 4.3). Myelin is a connective covering surrounding motor nerve axons and many sensory nerve axons. Myelin is produced by Schwann cells and functions to greatly increase the speed of nerve conduction. Myelin acts as an excellent insulator and permits saltatory conduction. This occurs when depolarization takes place only at the internodal regions. For this reason, myelinated axons have their voltage-dependent sodium channels concentrated around the nodes, with few in the internodal regions. This type of 'jumping' conduction, where time is not required to depolarize axons between the nodes, permits a greater than 10-fold increase in velocity.

Velocities in myelinated nerves range from 40 to 70 m/sec. Unmyelinated axons, in contrast, are much slower – in the range of 1–5 m/sec. Unmyelinated axons do not conduct through saltatory conduction but have voltage-dependent channels uniformly throughout the nerve. The speed of nerve conduction is largely contingent upon the amount of time it takes for voltage-dependent channels to open. As unmyelinated nerves have a far greater

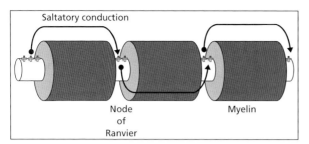

Figure 4.3
Myelinated nerve.

Saltatory conduction

Node
of
Ranvier

Myelin

number of channels per length of nerve, they conduct at less than one-tenth the speed of a myelinated nerve.

The most important points to remember about myelin are:

- Myelin helps nerves propagate an action potential faster.
- The myelin sheath functions as insulator of the axon.
- In myelinated nerves, depolarization occurs only at areas devoid of myelin (nodes of Ranvier) resulting in saltatory conduction.
- Conduction velocity is directly related to internodal length and efficiency of myelin insulation.

A demyelinated axon is a myelinated nerve that has lost its myelin covering. This does *not* become an unmyelinated nerve. While an unmyelinated axon can conduct an impulse along its entire length, a demyelinated axon may not be able to conduct across a demyelinated area. This loss of conduction across a lesion is referred to as *conduction block*. The term *neurapraxia* is used to describe a lesion where conduction block is present.

It is important to note that while axons have an 'all or none' response, an action potential represents the summation of many axons. Thus, a neurapraxic lesion can result in an amplitude decrement from less than 1% to nearly 100%. In reality, neurapraxic lesions of less than 20% are rarely diagnosed due to the amplitude differences normally seen from different sites of stimulation.

After a demyelinating lesion, as part of the recovery phase, there is typically regeneration of immature myelin. This immature myelin will not insulate as well as mature myelin and therefore during a NCS you may see a return of conduction but at a slower than normal velocity. *Therefore, conduction slowing and conduction block are indicative of demyelinating, but not axonal lesions.*

 ## The Action Potential

The action potential is a summation of many potentials. In a CMAP it is the summation of motor units (muscle fibers) that are firing, while a SNAP is a summation of individual nerve fibers, each with its own amplitude and slightly different conduction velocities. This summation yields a characteristic (usually bell-shaped) curve. The part of the curve that begins to rise first represents the components from the fastest fibers. The typical action potential is shown on a time versus amplitude chart (Fig. 4.4). The amplitude can be measured from onset to peak (A–B) or from peak to trough (B–C). The duration is the time from the onset to recovery (A–D). The area is the area under the negative phase of the potential. (In electrodiagnostic terminology, *negative* refers to an *upward* deflection from baseline and *positive* refers to a *downward* deflection from baseline.)

Figure 4.4
Compound
muscle action
potential.

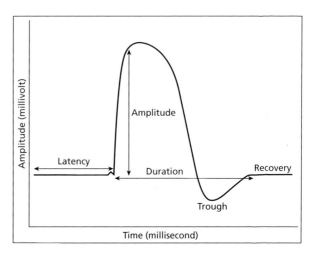

Components of the Action Potential

Latency

The *latency* represents the time it takes from stimulation of the nerve to the measurement of the beginning of the sensory nerve action potential (SNAP) or the compound muscle action potential (CMAP). In a CMAP, the *onset latency* represents the arrival time (at the pickup electrode over the muscle) of the fastest-conducting nerve fibers. There is normal variation in the conduction velocity of the individual nerve fibers producing a temporally dispersed curve. This is usually a gaussian or bell-shaped curve representing the number of fibers (amplitude) and how fast they are traveling (latency). The nerve fibers that contribute to the trough of the curve are amongst the slowest fibers.

In sensory nerves, the latency is solely dependent on the speed of conduction of the fastest fibers and the distance the wave of depolarization travels. In motor nerves, in addition to the speed of the nerve and the distance traveled, the latency is also dependent on the amount of time it takes to synapse at the neuromuscular junction and the speed of intramuscular conduction. While this is typically brief (estimated to be approximately one millisecond) the exact duration can vary. Usually the latency is measured to the negative (upward) departure from baseline. If an initial positive departure is seen, the electrodes usually require repositioning, because it is likely that the recording electrode is over a muscle not innervated by the nerve being stimulated.

It must be stressed that a latency measurement without a standardized or recorded distance is meaningless. For example, if a patient has a large hand, the standard distance of 8 cm for median motor latency may not allow you to stimulate above the wrist. If you stimulate at 10 cm, but don't record that you stimulated at a distance of 10 cm, it will appear that the patient has slowing of the median nerve across the wrist, because it will take longer to travel a further distance. Normal latencies are listed in Chapter 22.

Conduction Velocity

Conduction velocity is how fast the nerve is propagating an action potential. It can be calculated by the formula:

$$velocity = distance/time$$

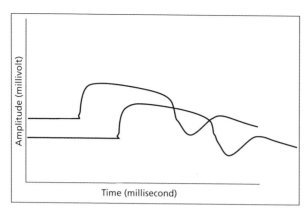

Figure 4.5
Temporal
dispersion

As stated above, sensory nerves do not have a myoneural junction. Therefore, conduction velocity can be calculated directly by measuring the time it takes (in milliseconds) for the propagated action potential to travel the measured distance (in centimeters). Since *motor nerves* do conduct across a myoneural junction, the conduction velocity cannot be measured directly. Therefore, we use the formula:

$$\text{velocity} = \text{change in distance/change in time}$$

At least two sites must be stimulated (the same nerve is stimulated both proximally and distally while recording over the same muscle). The difference in distance from the two stimulation sites is then divided by the difference in latencies of the two action potentials obtained. Normal conduction velocities average above 50 meters/second in the upper extremities and above 40 meters/second in the lower extremities.

Amplitude

The *amplitude* of a CMAP represents the sum of the amplitudes of individual potentials. These individual potentials are generated by muscle fibers that are depolarized by nerve fiber axons of similar conduction velocity. The *amplitude is therefore dependent on the integrity of the axons, the muscle fibers it depolarizes, and on the extent of variability of the conduction velocity of individual fibers*. If some fibers are slow and others are fast then the action potential will be of longer duration (temporal dispersion) and lower amplitude (Fig. 4.5). When there is a CMAP with low amplitude, it is important to distinguish whether this is occurring because of temporal dispersion or is due to decreased number of axons (Fig. 4.6).

The way you figure this out is that the duration of the action potential is prolonged in temporal dispersion and not prolonged if the amplitude is truly reduced. The area *under the curve* is an alternative way to estimate the number of axons/muscle fibers that are depolarized. In most cases, area measurements and amplitude measurements yield similar results and either is used in common practice. Motor nerve amplitudes are measured in millivolts. Sensory nerve amplitudes are much smaller and are measured in microvolts. *CMAP amplitude is most often measured from baseline to negative peak* or can be measured *peak-to-peak*. *SNAP amplitude is measured from negative peak to positive peak or baseline to negative peak*.

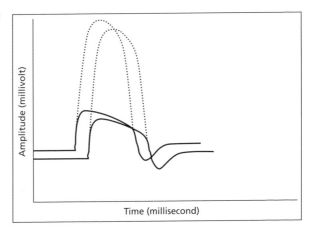

Figure 4.6 Axonal loss. Dotted line indicates normal amplitude.

Duration

The *duration* is the time from the onset latency to termination latency. In other words, the time from departure from baseline to final return to baseline. In some demyelinating diseases with nerve fibers affected differently, the duration may be increased (temporal dispersion). Generally, temporal dispersion is seen in acquired as opposed to congenital neuropathies.

Technical Aspects

Stimulators

Stimulators are normally two metal or felt pad electrodes placed between 1.5 to 3 cm apart. When stimulating, in most cases the cathode (black or negative pole) is placed *toward* the direction in which the nerve is to be stimulated. The potential sites for stimulation are reviewed later in this chapter. Conduction gel should be used to ensure electrical contact. This may need to be reapplied periodically.

Sites of Stimulation

In order to accurately stimulate a nerve, it is necessary to recall the nerve's anatomy. Given a strong enough impulse, any nerve can be stimulated. The more superficial the nerve, the easier (and more accurate) stimulation becomes. In reality, nerves are usually stimulated when they are relatively superficial. This permits an electrical impulse that the patient can tolerate. Superficial stimulation also allows a more precise localization of the site on the nerve where it is stimulated. The farther away the nerve is from the cathode the stronger the stimulus required. *Supramaximal stimulation* occurs when further increases in the intensity of the stimulus will not change the amplitude of the recorded potential. Increases beyond this point however, can change the latency or stimulate adjacent nerves. Care should be taken not to 'over stimulate'.

Some nerves may only be accessible to stimulation for a limited distance along the course of the nerve, whereas others can be stimulated at many sites along the nerve. In simple motor nerve studies usually two stimulus sites are used. In cases of suspected entrapment, it is important to be able to stimulate proximal and distal to the suspected area.

Recording Electrodes

Three electrodes are used to record a potential in nerve conduction studies and electromyography. They are the *active*, *reference* and *ground electrodes*.

Active electrode: The active electrode, also referred to as E1 or G1, should be placed over the muscle belly (preferably over the motor point, where the nerve enters the muscle) during motor studies. During sensory studies, the active electrode should be placed directly over the nerve (where the nerve is as superficial as possible).

Reference electrode: The reference electrode (sometimes called the E2 or G2) should be placed on a nearby tendon or bone *away* from the muscle when attempting to record a CMAP. When performing sensory nerve action potentials (SNAPS), it has been shown that 3–4 cm is the optimal inter-electrode separation. If SNAP electrodes are placed too close to each other, decreased amplitude resembling an axonal lesion can occur. Compound muscle action potentials (CMAP) are less affected than SNAPS when electrodes are placed less than 3–4 cm apart.

Ground electrode: The third type of electrode is called the ground electrode. Grounding is important for obtaining a response that is free of too much artifact. Usually the ground is larger than the recording electrodes and provides a large surface area in contact with the patient. The ground electrode should be placed *between* the stimulating electrode and the recording electrode.

Late Responses

The H-reflex is a monosynaptic or oligosynaptic spinal reflex involving both motor and sensory fibers. It electrically tests some of the same fibers as are tested in the ankle jerk reflexes. In fact it is rare to be unable to obtain an H-reflex in the presence of an ankle jerk reflex. If this occurs, technical factors should be considered. In theory it is a sensitive measure in assessing radiculopathy because 1. it helps to assess proximal lesions, 2. it becomes abnormal relatively early in the development of radiculopathy, and 3. it incorporates sensory fiber function proximal to the dorsal root ganglion. The H-reflex primarily assesses afferent and efferent S1 fibers. Clinically, L5 and S1 radiculopathies may appear similar on EMG due to the overlap of myotomes. H-reflexes are probably of greatest value in distinguishing S1 from L5 radiculopathies.

When assessing for S1 radiculopathy, the H-reflex latency is recorded from the gastrocnemius-soleus muscle group upon stimulating the tibial nerve in the popliteal fossa (Fig. 4.7). The H-reflex is elicited with a submaximal stimulation with the cathode proximal to the anode. As the intensity of the stimulation is gradually increased from peak H-amplitude, we generally see a diminishment of the H-amplitude with a concurrent increase in the M wave amplitude. With supra maximal stimulation, the H-reflex is usually absent.

The H-reflex can also be used in C6/C7 radiculopathy by recording over the flexor carpi radialis muscle and stimulating the median nerve at the elbow. The median H-reflex is less commonly performed and clinically is less likely to be helpful for radiculopathy than a lower extremity H-reflex. Generally, gastrocnemius-soleus H-reflex latency side-to-side differences of greater than 1.5 ms are suggestive of S1 radiculopathy.

Although the H-reflex is sensitive, it has certain limitations: 1. patients with S_1 radiculopathy can have a normal H-reflex; 2. an abnormal H-reflex is only suggestive, but not definitive for radiculopathy because the abnormality may originate in other components of the long pathway involved, such as the peripheral nerves, plexuses, or spinal cord; 3. once the H-reflex becomes abnormal, it usually does not return to normal,

Figure 4.7 Setup
for H-reflex

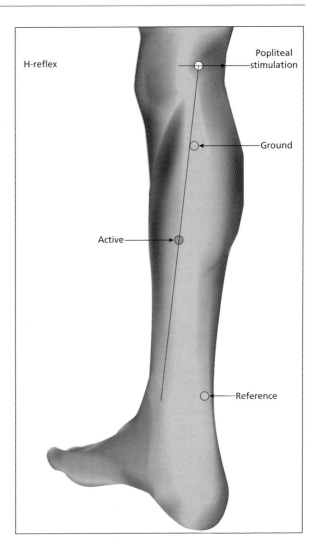

even over time; and finally the H-reflex is often absent in otherwise normal individuals over the age of 60 years. The reflexes therefore can be considered a sensitive, but not specific indicator of pathology. Latency of the H-reflex is dependent on the age and leg length of the patient (Table 4.1). A side-to-side amplitude difference of 60% or more may also indicate pathology.

F-waves are low amplitude late responses thought to be due to antidromic activation of motor neurons (anterior horn cells) following peripheral nerve stimulation, which then cause orthodromic impulses to pass back along the involved motor axons. Some electromyographers have called this a 'backfiring' of axons. It is called the F-wave because it was first noted in intrinsic foot muscles. The F-wave has small amplitude, a variable configuration, and a variable latency. Generally F-wave amplitudes are up to 5% of the orthodromically generated motor response (M-response). The most widely used

Table 4.1 H-reflex value based on the age and height: (H = 2.74 + 0.05 x age + 0.14 x height + 1.4)

Height (cm)	Age (years old)															
	15	20	25	30	35	40	45	50	55	60	65	70	75	80	85	90
100	18.89	19.14	19.39	19.64	19.89	20.14	20.39	20.64	20.89	21.14	21.39	21.64	21.89	22.14	22.39	22.64
110	20.29	20.54	20.79	21.04	21.29	21.54	21.79	22.04	22.29	22.54	22.79	23.04	23.29	23.54	23.79	24.04
120	21.69	21.94	22.19	22.44	22.69	22.94	23.19	23.44	23.69	23.94	24.19	24.44	24.69	24.94	25.19	25.44
130	23.09	23.34	23.59	23.84	24.09	24.34	24.59	24.84	25.09	25.34	25.59	25.84	26.09	26.34	26.59	26.84
135	23.79	24.04	24.29	24.54	24.79	25.04	25.29	25.54	25.79	26.04	26.29	26.54	26.79	27.04	27.29	27.54
140	24.49	24.74	24.99	25.24	25.49	25.74	25.99	26.24	26.49	26.74	26.99	27.24	27.49	27.74	27.99	28.24
141	24.63	24.88	25.13	25.38	25.63	25.88	26.13	26.38	26.63	26.88	27.13	27.38	27.63	27.88	28.13	28.38
142	24.77	25.02	25.27	25.52	25.77	26.02	26.27	26.52	26.77	27.02	27.27	27.52	27.77	28.02	28.27	28.52
143	24.91	25.16	25.41	25.66	25.91	26.16	26.41	26.66	26.91	27.16	27.41	27.66	27.91	28.16	28.41	28.66
144	25.05	25.3	25.55	25.8	26.05	26.3	26.55	26.8	27.05	27.3	27.55	27.8	28.05	28.3	28.55	28.8
145	25.19	25.44	25.69	25.94	26.19	26.44	26.69	26.94	27.19	27.44	27.69	27.94	28.19	28.44	28.69	28.94
146	25.33	25.58	25.83	26.08	26.33	26.58	26.83	27.08	27.33	27.58	27.83	28.08	28.33	28.58	28.83	29.08
147	25.47	25.72	25.97	26.22	26.47	26.72	26.97	27.22	27.47	27.72	27.97	28.22	28.47	28.72	28.97	29.22
148	25.61	25.86	26.11	26.36	26.61	26.86	27.11	27.36	27.61	27.86	28.11	28.36	28.61	28.86	29.11	29.36
149	25.75	26	26.25	26.5	26.75	27	27.25	27.5	27.75	28	28.25	28.5	28.75	29	29.25	29.5
150	25.89	26.14	26.39	26.64	26.89	27.14	27.39	27.64	27.89	28.14	28.39	28.64	28.89	29.14	29.39	29.64
151	26.03	26.28	26.53	26.78	27.03	27.28	27.53	27.78	28.03	28.28	28.53	28.78	29.03	29.28	29.53	29.78
152	26.17	26.42	26.67	26.92	27.17	27.42	27.67	27.92	28.17	28.42	28.67	28.92	29.17	29.42	29.67	29.92
153	26.31	26.56	26.81	27.06	27.31	27.56	27.81	28.06	28.31	28.56	28.81	29.06	29.31	29.56	29.81	30.06
154	26.45	26.7	26.95	27.2	27.45	27.7	27.95	28.2	28.45	28.7	28.95	29.2	29.45	29.7	29.95	30.2
155	26.59	26.84	27.09	27.34	27.59	27.84	28.09	28.34	28.59	28.84	29.09	29.34	29.59	29.84	30.09	30.34
156	26.73	26.98	27.23	27.48	27.73	27.98	28.23	28.48	28.73	28.98	29.23	29.48	29.73	29.98	30.23	30.48

Table 4.1 H-reflex value based on the age and height: (H = 2.74 + 0.05 × age + 0.14 × height + 1.4) *(cont'd)*

Height (cm)	Age (years old)															
	15	20	25	30	35	40	45	50	55	60	65	70	75	80	85	90
157	26.87	27.12	27.37	27.62	27.87	28.12	28.37	28.62	28.87	29.12	29.37	29.62	29.87	30.12	30.37	30.62
158	27.01	27.26	27.51	27.76	28.01	28.26	28.51	28.76	29.01	29.26	29.51	29.76	30.01	30.26	30.51	30.76
159	27.15	27.4	27.65	27.9	28.15	28.4	28.65	28.9	29.15	29.4	29.65	29.9	30.15	30.4	30.65	30.9
160	27.29	27.54	27.79	28.04	28.29	28.54	28.79	29.04	29.29	29.54	29.79	30.04	30.29	30.54	30.79	31.04
161	27.43	27.68	27.93	28.18	28.43	28.68	28.93	29.18	29.43	29.68	29.93	30.18	30.43	30.68	30.93	31.18
162	27.57	27.82	28.07	28.32	28.57	28.82	29.07	29.32	29.57	29.82	30.07	30.32	30.57	30.82	31.07	31.32
163	27.71	27.96	28.21	28.46	28.71	28.96	29.21	29.46	29.71	29.96	30.21	30.46	30.71	30.96	31.21	31.46
164	27.85	28.1	28.35	28.6	28.85	29.1	29.35	29.6	29.85	30.1	30.35	30.6	30.85	31.1	31.35	31.6
165	27.99	28.24	28.49	28.74	28.99	29.24	29.49	29.74	29.99	30.24	30.49	30.74	30.99	31.24	31.49	31.74
166	28.13	28.38	28.63	28.88	29.13	29.38	29.63	29.88	30.13	30.38	30.63	30.88	31.13	31.38	31.63	31.88
167	28.27	28.52	28.77	29.02	29.27	29.52	29.77	30.02	30.27	30.52	30.77	31.02	31.27	31.52	31.77	32.02
168	28.41	28.66	28.91	29.16	29.41	29.66	29.91	30.16	30.41	30.66	30.91	31.16	31.41	31.66	31.91	32.16
169	28.55	28.8	29.05	29.3	29.55	29.8	30.05	30.3	30.55	30.8	31.05	31.3	31.55	31.8	32.05	32.3
170	28.69	28.94	29.19	29.44	29.69	29.94	30.19	30.44	30.69	30.94	31.19	31.44	31.69	31.94	32.19	32.44
171	28.83	29.08	29.33	29.58	29.83	30.08	30.33	30.58	30.83	31.08	31.33	31.58	31.83	32.08	32.33	32.58
172	28.97	29.22	29.47	29.72	29.97	30.22	30.47	30.72	30.97	31.22	31.47	31.72	31.97	32.22	32.47	32.72
173	29.11	29.36	29.61	29.86	30.11	30.36	30.61	30.86	31.11	31.36	31.61	31.86	32.11	32.36	32.61	32.86
174	29.25	29.5	29.75	30	30.25	30.5	30.75	31	31.25	31.5	31.75	32	32.25	32.5	32.75	33
175	29.39	29.64	29.89	30.14	30.39	30.64	30.89	31.14	31.39	31.64	31.89	32.14	32.39	32.64	32.89	33.14
176	29.53	29.78	30.03	30.28	30.53	30.78	31.03	31.28	31.53	31.78	32.03	32.28	32.53	32.78	33.03	33.28
177	29.67	29.92	30.17	30.42	30.67	30.92	31.17	31.42	31.67	31.92	32.17	32.42	32.67	32.92	33.17	33.42
178	29.81	30.06	30.31	30.56	30.81	31.06	31.31	31.56	31.81	32.06	32.31	32.56	32.81	33.06	33.31	33.56

Table 4.1 H-reflex value based on the age and height: (H = 2.74 + 0.05 × age + 0.14 × height + 1.4) (cont'd)

Height (cm)	Age (years old)															
	15	20	25	30	35	40	45	50	55	60	65	70	75	80	85	90
179	29.95	30.2	30.45	30.7	30.95	31.2	31.45	31.7	31.95	32.2	32.45	32.7	32.95	33.2	33.45	33.7
180	30.09	30.34	30.59	30.84	31.09	31.34	31.59	31.84	32.09	32.34	32.59	32.84	33.09	33.34	33.59	33.84
181	30.23	30.48	30.73	30.98	31.23	31.48	31.73	31.98	32.23	32.48	32.73	32.98	33.23	33.48	33.73	33.98
182	30.37	30.62	30.87	31.12	31.37	31.62	31.87	32.12	32.37	32.62	32.87	33.12	33.37	33.62	33.87	34.12
183	30.51	30.76	31.01	31.26	31.51	31.76	32.01	32.26	32.51	32.76	33.01	33.26	33.51	33.76	34.01	34.26
184	30.65	30.9	31.15	31.4	31.65	31.9	32.15	32.4	32.65	32.9	33.15	33.4	33.65	33.9	34.15	34.4
185	30.79	31.04	31.29	31.54	31.79	32.04	32.29	32.54	32.79	33.04	33.29	33.54	33.79	34.04	34.29	34.54
186	30.93	31.18	31.43	31.68	31.93	32.18	32.43	32.68	32.93	33.18	33.43	33.68	33.93	34.18	34.43	34.68
187	31.07	31.32	31.57	31.82	32.07	32.32	32.57	32.82	33.07	33.32	33.57	33.82	34.07	34.32	34.57	34.82
188	31.21	31.46	31.71	31.96	32.21	32.46	32.71	32.96	33.21	33.46	33.71	33.96	34.21	34.46	34.71	34.96
189	31.35	31.6	31.85	32.1	32.35	32.6	32.85	33.1	33.35	33.6	33.85	34.1	34.35	34.6	34.85	35.1
190	31.49	31.74	31.99	32.24	32.49	32.74	32.99	33.24	33.49	33.74	33.99	34.24	34.49	34.74	34.99	35.24
191	31.63	31.88	32.13	32.38	32.63	32.88	33.13	33.38	33.63	33.88	34.13	34.38	34.63	34.88	35.13	35.38
192	31.77	32.02	32.27	32.52	32.77	33.02	33.27	33.52	33.77	34.02	34.27	34.52	34.77	35.02	35.27	35.52
193	31.91	32.16	32.41	32.66	32.91	33.16	33.41	33.66	33.91	34.16	34.41	34.66	34.91	35.16	35.41	35.66
194	32.05	32.3	32.55	32.8	33.05	33.3	33.55	33.8	34.05	34.3	34.55	34.8	35.05	35.3	35.55	35.8
195	32.19	32.44	32.69	32.94	33.19	33.44	33.69	33.94	34.19	34.44	34.69	34.94	35.19	35.44	35.69	35.94
196	32.33	32.58	32.83	33.08	33.33	33.58	33.83	34.08	34.33	34.58	34.83	35.08	35.33	35.58	35.83	36.08
197	32.47	32.72	32.97	33.22	33.47	33.72	33.97	34.22	34.47	34.72	34.97	35.22	35.47	35.72	35.97	36.22
198	32.61	32.86	33.11	33.36	33.61	33.86	34.11	34.36	34.61	34.86	35.11	35.36	35.61	35.86	36.11	36.36
199	32.75	33	33.25	33.5	33.75	34	34.25	34.5	34.75	35	35.25	35.5	35.75	36	36.25	36.5
200	32.89	33.14	33.39	33.64	33.89	34.14	34.39	34.64	34.89	35.14	35.39	35.64	35.89	36.14	36.39	36.64

Table 4.1 H-reflex value based on the age and height: ($H = 2.74 + 0.05 \times age + 0.14 \times height + 1.4$) (cont'd)

Height (cm)	Age (years old)															
	15	20	25	30	35	40	45	50	55	60	65	70	75	80	85	90
201	33.03	33.28	33.53	33.78	34.03	34.28	34.53	34.78	35.03	35.28	35.53	35.78	36.03	36.28	36.53	36.78
202	33.17	33.42	33.67	33.92	34.17	34.42	34.67	34.92	35.17	35.42	35.67	35.92	36.17	36.42	36.67	36.92
203	33.31	33.56	33.81	34.06	34.31	34.56	34.81	35.06	35.31	35.56	35.81	36.06	36.31	36.56	36.81	37.06
204	33.45	33.7	33.95	34.2	34.45	34.7	34.95	35.2	35.45	35.7	35.95	36.2	36.45	36.7	36.95	37.2
205	33.59	33.84	34.09	34.34	34.59	34.84	35.09	35.34	35.59	35.84	36.09	36.34	36.59	36.84	37.09	37.34
206	33.73	33.98	34.23	34.48	34.73	34.98	35.23	35.48	35.73	35.98	36.23	36.48	36.73	36.98	37.23	37.48
207	33.73	33.98	34.23	34.48	34.73	34.98	35.23	35.48	35.73	35.98	36.23	36.48	36.73	36.98	37.23	37.48
208	34.01	34.26	34.51	34.76	35.01	35.26	35.51	35.76	36.01	36.26	36.51	36.76	37.01	37.26	37.51	37.76
209	34.15	34.4	34.65	34.9	35.15	35.4	35.65	35.9	36.15	36.4	36.65	36.9	37.15	37.4	37.65	37.9
210	34.29	34.54	34.79	35.04	35.29	35.54	35.79	36.04	36.29	36.54	36.79	37.04	37.29	37.54	37.79	38.04
215	34.99	35.24	35.49	35.74	35.99	36.24	36.49	36.74	36.99	37.24	37.49	37.74	37.99	38.24	38.49	38.74
220	35.69	35.94	36.19	36.44	36.69	36.94	37.19	37.44	37.69	37.94	38.19	38.44	38.69	38.94	39.19	39.44
230	37.09	37.34	37.59	37.84	38.09	38.34	38.59	38.84	39.09	39.34	39.59	39.84	40.09	40.34	40.59	40.84

parameter is the latency of the shortest reproducible response. The F-wave can be found in many muscles of the upper and lower extremities. Unfortunately F-waves have not turned out to be as sensitive a test as initially hoped. The reasons for this are:

1. the pathways involve only the motor fibers,
2. as with the H-reflex, it involves a long neuronal pathway so that if there is a focal lesion it might be obscured,
3. if an abnormality is present, the F-wave will not pinpoint the exact location because any lesion, from the anterior horn cell to the muscle being tested, can affect the F-wave similarly,
4. since muscles have multiple root innervations, the shortest latency may reflect the healthy fibers in the non-affected root, and
5. the latency and amplitude of an F-wave is variable so that multiple stimulations must be performed to find the shortest latency. If not enough stimulations are done (usually more than 10), the shortest latency may not be apparent. Thus, use of F-waves in evaluating for radiculopathy are extremely limited and should not be the sole basis upon which the diagnosis is made. See Table 4.2 for a comparison of H-reflex and F-waves.

F-wave Ratio

Because errors can occur when measuring distances for F-wave conduction velocities, an alternative F-wave technique was developed which did not require distance measurements. The ratio is as follows:

$$\frac{(\text{F-wave latency} - \text{CMAP latency}) - 1 \text{ ms}}{\text{CMAP latency} \times 2}$$

(M = CMAP latency; this ratio may be rewritten as $(F - M - 1)/2 M$). The ratio assumes that the distance from the elbow (or knee) to the hand (or foot) is approximately equal to the distance from the elbow (or knee) to the spinal cord (Fig. 4.8). Therefore, stimulation must be performed at the elbow or knee.

The normal F-wave ratio in the upper limb is approximately 1 ± 0.3 and in the lower limb the normal F-ratio is 1.1 ± 0.3. A ratio higher than 1.3 indicates a proximal lesion, since the numerator of the equation includes the proximal stimulation from the F-wave. A ratio below 0.7 indicates a distal lesion, since a larger CMAP latency will decrease the numerator and increase the denominator. Therefore, an F-ratio is not necessarily more sensitive than F-latency, but it does allow one to assess whether the slowing is in the proximal or distal segment of the nerve. It should be noted that F-waves are non-specific. Therefore, interpreting NCS results using F-waves must be done in conjunction with other information.

Important Points to Remember

- When stimulating proximal and distal sites, the waveforms should be similar in morphology and duration. For motor studies, amplitude should not decrease by more than 20% on proximal stimulation (when compared to the distal amplitude).
- Non-identical waveforms may be secondary to accidental stimulation of another nerve. For example, the peroneal and tibial nerves are very close in the popliteal fossa. If the *pulse width* (duration of the stimulus) is increased, the wrong nerve may be stimulated. Usually, the CMAP that results will have an initial positive (downward)

Table 4.2 Comparison of H-reflex and F-wave

Parameter	H-reflex	F-wave
Derivation of name	Originally described by Hoffman	Originally obtained in foot muscles
Type of synapse	Monosynaptic or oligosynaptic	Polysynaptic
Pathway	Sensory orthodromic Motor antidromic	Motor antidromic Motor orthodromic
Stimulus required	Submaximal (stronger stimulation produces inhibition secondary to collision of orthodromic impulses by antidromic conduction in motor axons)	Supramaximal
Where they can be elicited? (Normals)	Soleus Flexor carpi radialis	Most muscles (distal preferred)
Stimulation site	Posterior tibial nerve in popliteal fossa	Along peripheral nerve
Stimulus cathode	Proximal	Proximal
Size of response (compared to M)	Amplification of motor response centrally (due to reflex activation of motor neurons)	Small (motor neurons are activated infrequently with antidromic stimulation)
Facilitation	Enhanced by maneuvers that increase motor-neuron pool excitability (contraction or CNS lesion)	N/A
Uses	S_1 Radiculopathy (sensitive but not specific) Guillain–Barré syndrome	Demyelinating polyneuropathies Guillain–Barré Proximal nerve or root injury (not test of choice – non-specific)
Latency, amplitude and configuration	Reproducible latency and configuration (amplitude dependent on stimulation)	Variable in amplitude, latency and configuration
Side-to-side difference	> 1.5 msec	>2 msec from hand >3 msec from calf >4 msec from foot
Ratio	N/A	$\dfrac{F - M - 1}{2\,M}$

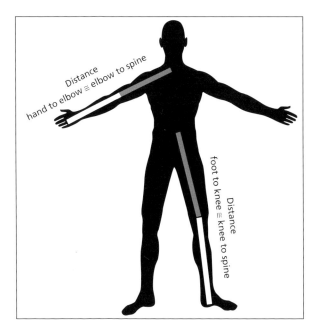

Figure 4.8 F-wave ratios are calculated based on the assumption that the distance from the elbow (or knee) to the hand (or foot) is approximately equal to the distance from the elbow (or knee) to the spinal cord

deflection, since the active electrode is not over the muscle being stimulated. (If you are not sure which nerve is being stimulated, check for the physiological response. For example, if the ankle plantar flexes, the tibial nerve is usually being stimulated.)

- An increased duration (and smaller amplitude) on proximal stimulation could indicate a segmental demyelination in the segment being stimulated. In this situation (referred to as temporal dispersion), the area under the curve of the CMAP should not change. All of the axons are still contributing to the CMAP, but some are conducting much slower than others (see Fig. 4.8).

- A decrease of more than 20% amplitude with the proximal stimulation (compared to the distal amplitude) could indicate a conduction block across the segment. A conduction block occurs when an area of demyelination is so severe that saltatory conduction cannot occur. The impulse is 'blocked' from propagating and therefore those axons cannot help to contribute to the amplitude of the CMAP. Remember, however, that this is a focal myelin problem, not an axonal problem, even though the amplitude is affected.

- With motor nerves, a distance of at least 10 cm between stimulation points should be used in order to decrease the likelihood of a measurement error significantly affecting the calculated conduction velocity. Since velocity = distance/time, a 1 cm error in measuring over a 5-cm distance will result in a 20% error in distance and will significantly affect the calculated conduction velocity. If the distance is 10 cm, a 1 cm error only results in a 10% error in distance. Generally, due to skin elasticity and other factors, a measurement will be accurate to within about 1 cm. Obesity in the patient may decrease the ability to accurately measure the length of the nerve segment.

- You can estimate the amount of axonal loss in an acute peripheral nerve lesion if you compare the amplitude of the CMAP on the unaffected side. For example, if the

Table 4.3 Nerve conduction studies setup

Nerve	Active electrode	Reference electrode	Ground	Stimulation
MEDIAN – *Motor* (see Fig. A1.1)	Place on the anatomic center of the abductor pollicis brevis. (Usually about ½ the distance from the distal wrist crease to the metacarpal phalangeal joint.)	Place on the proximal phalanx of the thumb. Place 3–4 cm distal to the recording electrode	Placed on the dorsum of the hand between the active electrode and the stimulator	1. *Midwrist:* Distal stimulation is on the palmar surface of the hand between the tendons of the flexor carpi radialis and the palmaris longus. Stimulation should be 8 cm proximal to the active electrode. 2. *Elbow:* Stimulate proximal and medial to the antecubital space, just lateral to the brachial artery. 3. *Axilla:* Stimulation is performed in the axilla at least 10 cm proximal to the elbow stimulation
MEDIAN – *Sensory (Orthodromic)* (see Fig. A1.2)	Place 14 cm proximal from the ring cathode at the midwrist. (This should be about the same spot where the motor portion was stimulated.)	Place 3–4 cm proximal to the recording electrode	Place on the dorsum of the hand between the stimulating ring electrodes and the recording electrode	Since this is in the physiological direction, stimulate distally from the 2nd digit using ring electrodes. *Ring cathode:* The cathode is placed near the PIP joint. *Ring anode:* Place around the second DIP

Table 4.3 Nerve conduction studies setup (*cont'd*)

Nerve	Active electrode	Reference electrode	Ground	Stimulation
MEDIAN – *Sensory (Antidromic)* (see Fig. A1.3)	Place over the proximal interphalangeal joint on the 2nd finger	Place the reference electrode over the distal interphalangeal joint	Ground is placed on the dorsum of the hand between the active electrode and stimulator	The stimulation points occur: 7 cm proximal to the active electrode at the mid palm, and 7 cm proximal to the mid palm at the wrist (between the tendons of the flexor carpi radialis and the palmaris longus). (For large hands, 8 cm can be used. For small hands, 6 cm can be used.)
ULNAR – *motor* (see Fig. A1.4)	Place on the center of the abductor digiti minimi. It may help to palpate that muscle by abducting the 5th digit	Place distally over the 5th digit	Place on the dorsum of the hand between the active and stimulating electrode	1. *Wrist:* stimulate 8 cm proximally from the active electrode. This is usually just medial to the flexor carpi ulnaris tendon. 2. *Below the elbow:* when stimulating at the elbow region, you must flex the elbow so there is an angle of about 90 degrees. Feel for the ulnar groove (the funny bone) and stimulate just below this area.

Table 4.3 Nerve conduction studies setup (*cont'd*)

Nerve	Active electrode	Reference electrode	Ground	Stimulation
				3. *Above the elbow:* Stimulation site is located at least 10 cm proximal to the below elbow stimulation in line with the path of the ulnar nerve. 4. *Axilla:* This stimulation site is located at least 10 cm proximal to the above elbow site at about the midpoint of the arm in the axilla
Remember that the arm should be maintained with the same elbow flexion when stimulating and measuring the nerve. The responses from all four sites should be similar in waveform, amplitude and duration.				
Dorsal ulnar cutaneous nerve (see Fig. A1.5)	On the dorsum of the hand, between the fourth and fifth metacarpal bones	Base of the 5th digit	Place on the dorsum of the hand between the active and stimulating electrode	14 cm proximal to the active electrode, between the ulna and the flexor carpi ulnaris muscle
ULNAR *sensory (orthodromic)* (see Fig A1.6)	Place 14 cm proximally from the stimulating ring cathode on the ulnar side of the wrist	Position 3–4 cm proximal to the active electrode	Place on the dorsum of the hand between the stimulating and recording electrodes	*Ring cathode:* Place over the PIP joint of the 5th finger. *Ring anode:* Place over the 5th DIP joint

Table 4.3 Nerve conduction studies setup (*cont'd*)

Nerve	Active electrode	Reference electrode	Ground	Stimulation
ULNAR *sensory* *(antidromic)* (see Fig. A1.7)	Place on the 5th digit over the PIP joint	Place over the 5th DIP joint, so that a distance of not less than 3 cm is maintained	Place on the dorsum of the hand between the active and stimulating electrodes	Stimulate at the wrist a distance of 14 cm proximal from the active electrode near the proximal crease of the wrist
RADIAL *sensory* *(antidromic)* (see Fig. A1.8)	Place over the sensory branch as it crosses the extensor pollicis longus tendon. Can be palpated on ulnar side of the anatomic snuffbox when the thumb is extended	Place on the lateral side of the head of the 2nd metacarpal about 3–4 cm distal to the active electrode	Place between the active electrode and the stimulating site	Stimulate 10–14 cm proximal to the active electrode over the radial side of the forearm
Alternative Radial Sensory *(antidromic)* (see Fig. A1.8)	Ring electrode over the metacarpal phalangeal joint of the thumb	Ring electrode over the interphalangeal joint of the thumb	Place on the dorsum of the hand	Stimulate 11 cm proximal to the active electrode, in the anatomical snuffbox
RADIAL *motor* (see Fig. A1.9)	Place over the extensor indicis proprius on the dorsum of the hand. Locate by extending the 2nd digit. (A needle is sometimes used instead of a surface electrode.) Note that the amplitude of the CMAP cannot be compared if using a needle for the active electrode	Place over the ulnar styloid	Place between the active electrode and the stimulation site	*Forearm:* 8 cm proximal to the ulnar styloid just radial to the extensor carpi ulnaris muscle. *Elbow:* Stimulate 6 cm distal to the lateral epicondyle of the humerus (which is between the biceps tendon and the brachio-radialis muscle.)

Table 4.3 Nerve conduction studies setup (*cont'd*)

Nerve	Active electrode	Reference electrode	Ground	Stimulation
				Axilla: stimulate at the medial edge of the triceps with the arm externally rotated and the forearm supinated
LATERAL ANTEBRACHIAL CUTANEOUS *antidromic sensory* (see Fig. A1.10)	Draw a line from the stimulation point to the radial styloid. Place the reference electrode 12 cm distal to the cathode along this line	Place the reference electrode 4 cm distal to the active electrode	Place between the active electrode and the stimulation site	The cathode is placed at the elbow crease lateral to the biceps tendon
MUSCULO-CUTANEOUS *Motor* (see Fig. A1.11)	Place just distal to the midportion of the biceps muscle	Place just proximal to the antecubital fossa, where the biceps tendon meets the muscle fibers	Place over the deltoid muscle	The cathode is placed above the upper clavicle and lateral to the sternoclei-domastoid muscle. The anode is placed superiorly to the cathode (Erb's point)
AXILLARY Motor (see Fig. A1.12)	Place on the middle of the deltoid muscle	Place over the insertion of the deltoid on the lateral surface of the humerus	Place between the active electrode and the stimulation site	The cathode is placed lateral to where the sternoclei-domastoid muscle meets the clavicle, just above the clavicle. The anode is placed superiorly and angled medially (Erb's point)

Table 4.3 Nerve conduction studies setup (*cont'd*)

Nerve	Active electrode	Reference electrode	Ground	Stimulation
PERONEAL* (see Fig. A1.13)	Place on the anatomic center of the extensor digitorum brevis (EDB). Ask the patient to extend their toes and palpate for the muscle on the anterior lateral surface on the dorsum of the foot (usually located about 6 cm from the lateral malleolus.)	Place on the 5th toe	Place between the active electrode and the stimulation site	*Ankle:* Measure 8 cm proximal to the EDB on the lateral anterior surface of the foot. *Fibula:* Stimulate below the head of the fibula anterior to the neck of the fibula. *Popliteal:* Measure at least 10 cm proximal from the fibula and stimulate in the lateral border of the popliteal fossa. Look for ankle dorsiflexion
Sural – *sensory* (see Fig. A1.14)	Line up the active electrode inferior to the lateral malleolus (about 2 cm) and make sure it is parallel to the sole of the foot	Place distal (at least 3 cm) to the active electrode and parallel to the sole of the foot	Place between the active electrode and the stimulation site	Measure 14 cm proximal from the active electrode near the midline of the gastroc-nemius. Work your way laterally until an acceptable SNAP is achieved

* Note: In many normal individuals, the EDB muscle may be atrophied. If low amplitude is obtained, it may be useful to place the active electrode over the tibialis anterior muscle and stimulate at the fibular head.

Table 4.3 Nerve conduction studies setup (*cont'd*)

Nerve	Active electrode	Reference electrode	Ground	Stimulation
Posterior Tibial 1 – *motor* (see Fig. A1.15)	Place on the abductor hallucis muscle. Feel for the navicular bone of the foot and go 1 fingerbreadth toward the plantar surface of the foot and 1 fingerbreadth toward the great toe	Place on the great toe's medial surface	Place between the active electrode and the stimulation site	1. Go slightly posterior to the medial malleolus and stimulate 10 cm proximal to the active electrode. 2. Stimulate in the popliteal fossa, slightly lateral to its midline. (Look for ankle plantar flexion with stimulation.)
SUPERFICIAL PERONEAL SENSORY (see Fig. A1.16)	Place about one fingerbreadth medial to the lateral malleolus	Place at least 3 cm distal to the active electrode	Place on the anterior tibia between the active electrode and the stimulation site	Stimulate 14 cm proximal to the active electrode along the anterior and lateral surface of the leg
SCIATIC (see Fig. A1.17)	Place on the EDB muscle (peroneal component) or abductor hallucis muscle (tibial component)	Place on the small toe (peroneal comp.) or great toe (tibial comp.)	Place ground on the dorsum of the foot	Stimulate using a needle in the middle of the gluteal fold
LATERAL FEMORAL CUTANEOUS – *Antidromic* (see Fig. A1.18)	Draw a line from the ASIS to the lateral border of the patella. Place the active electrode 16–18 cm distally along this line	Place the reference electrode about 3 cm distal to the reference electrode along the same line connecting the ASIS and the lateral patella	Place between the active electrode and the stimulation site	Stimulate 1 cm medial to the ASIS. If using a cathode needle for stimulation, place a monopolar needle 1 cm medial to the ASIS, and place the anode several centimeters proximal

Table 4.3 Nerve conduction studies setup (*cont'd*)

Nerve	Active electrode	Reference electrode	Ground	Stimulation
H-REFLEX (see Fig. A1.19)	Measure the distance between the popliteal crease and the medial malleolus. Place the active electrode halfway between the above measured distances. (Over the medial gastrocnemius muscle.)	Place on the Achilles tendon	Place between the active electrode and the stimulation site	Stimulate in the popliteal fossa, slightly lateral to the midline. Remember to turn the stimulator around with the cathode proximal to the anode. A stimulus just greater than that to evoke a minimal M response is applied to the posterior tibial nerve in the center of the popliteal crease
F-WAVE	Same setup used for motor nerve conduction of individual nerves			Position the cathode proximal and use a supra-maximal stimulus to the nerve using standard electrode placements

amplitude of a median CMAP is 10 millivolts on the non-affected side, and 5 millivolts on the affected side, you can estimate that approximately 50% of the axons have been lost.

● When stimulating the ulnar nerve, the elbow should be bent to 70–90 degrees. If the elbow is held straight, the calculated conduction velocity will be falsely decreased. However the most important thing to remember is that if both elbows are not in the same position, there will be a false side-to-side velocity difference.

Table 4.3 includes, in chart form with illustrations, the proper placement of electrodes for the most commonly used motor and sensory studies. For the normal values of most peripheral nerve studies, see Chapter 22.

5

Electromyography

Lyn Weiss, Jay Weiss, Walter Gaudino, Victor Isaac, Kristin Gustafson

Electromyographic (EMG) testing involves evaluation of the electrical activity of a muscle and is one of the fundamental parts of the electrodiagnostic medical consultation. It is both an art and a science. It requires a thorough knowledge of the anatomy of the muscles being tested, machine settings and the neurophysiology behind the testing.

The electromyographer must be cognizant that the test is inherently uncomfortable. It is important to obtain the confidence and cooperation of the patient. Most patients are more comfortable when time is taken to explain the reasons for the testing and what information can be gained from the testing. It is a fallacy that the test is not uncomfortable and any attempt to convince a patient to the contrary is certain to fail. Some things that can be done to allay the patient's fear are to perform the study in a quiet room, speaking in a confident and calming manner, playing music of the patient's choice and keeping the room temperature comfortable.

Muscle Physiology

EMG assesses skeletal or voluntary muscle (rather than smooth or cardiac muscle). The muscle fibers that account for the strength of a contraction are extrafusal fibers (as opposed to intrafusal fibers of the muscle spindle). The extrafusal fibers are relaxed at rest with an intracellular resting potential of approximately –80 mV (similar to nerve fibers). The sarcolemma is a plasma membrane surrounding a muscle fiber. The action potential from a motor nerve fiber will synapse at the neuromuscular junction and then propagate along the sarcolemma. The sarcolemma has extensions into the muscle fibers called t-tubules. The depolarization of the t-tubules causes release of calcium from the sarcoplasmic reticulum. The calcium release results in changes in the actin and myosin. This shortens the actin-myosin functional unit, resulting in muscle contraction. EMG is actually measuring the electrical excitation of the muscle fibers.

Motor Units

Muscles contract and produce movement through the orderly recruitment of motor units. A *motor unit* is defined as one anterior horn cell, its axon, and all the muscle fibers innervated by that motor neuron. A motor unit is the fundamental structure that is assessed in electromyography. *The motor unit architecture* refers to its size, distribution, and endplate area. When a person starts to contract a muscle, the first motor units to fire are usually the smallest. These are the Type I motor units. As the contraction increases, there is an orderly recruitment of larger motor units (which have a higher threshold). They begin to fire and add to the force of the contraction.

Before You Begin

Most students of electrodiagnostic medicine are a little intimidated by the EMG part of the test. Sometimes, practicing with an orange can help you get the feel of the needle and how to position it. The 'feel' of transitioning the needle between the rind and the pulp of an orange is similar to piercing the muscle after inserting the needle through the skin. In keeping with the first tenet of medicine, 'first do no harm', it is important to know where to place the needle and why you are testing a certain muscle so as not to subject the patient to unnecessary testing. A good working knowledge of muscle anatomy is an essential tool for placing the needle in the appropriate muscle.

Electrodes

Just as with nerve conduction studies, you need a ground, a reference and an active electrode. The needle is the 'active electrode'; the reference may be separate or part of the needle itself. If the reference is separate it should be placed over the same muscle that is being tested by the needle. The ground can be placed anywhere on the extremity being tested.

Universal precautions must always be practiced during the needle portion of the test. This is to protect you as well as the patient. Universal precautions include using gloves, proper needle disposal, and using a one-handed technique for needle recapping. This can be done by securing the needle cap to the preamplifier and using one hand to place the needle back in the cap between muscle testing (Fig. 5.1).

Types of Needle Electrodes

Monopolar Needle

Monopolar needles are made of stainless steel and have a fine point insulated except at the distal 0.2 to 0.4 mm segment (Fig. 5.2). They require a surface electrode or a second needle in the subcutaneous tissue as a reference lead. A separate surface electrode placed on the skin serves as a ground. A monopolar needle records the voltage changes between the tip of the electrode and the reference. It registers a larger potential than a concentric needle using the same source. The reasons for this include the concentric needle's shape, picking up from a 180-degree field, whereas the monopolar picks up from a full 360-degree field around the needle. These differences in configuration help explain the larger amplitudes and increased polyphasicity recorded when a monopolar needle is used. A monopolar needle also has a smaller diameter and a teflon or similar coating. This makes the monopolar less uncomfortable than a concentric needle. This, combined with its cost advantage over the concentric, has led to its preferential clinical use.

Standard or Concentric Needle

A concentric needle is a stainless steel cannula similar to a hypodermic needle with a wire in the center of the shaft (Fig. 5.3). The pointed tip of the needle has an oval shape. While the wire is bare at the tip, the shaft can conduct electrical activity along its entire length. The needle, when near a source of electrical activity, registers the potential difference between the wire and the shaft. It is important to remember that the exposed active electrode is on the beveled portion of the cannula and thus is picking up from one direction (180 degrees rather than 360 degrees as in a monopolar needle). A separate surface electrode serves as the ground. The concentric electrode is less 'noisy' than the monopolar electrode, providing a clearer signal.

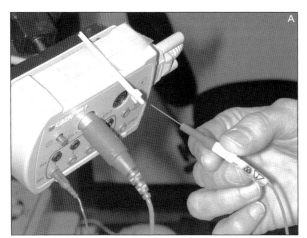

Figure 5.1 Needle recapping.

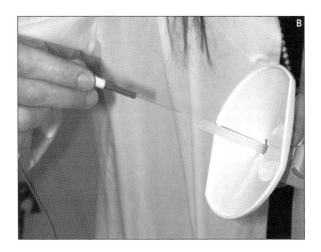

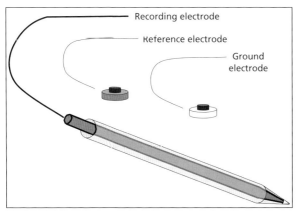

Figure 5.2 Monopolar needle.

Recording electrode

Reference electrode

Ground electrode

Figure 5.3
Concentric
needle.

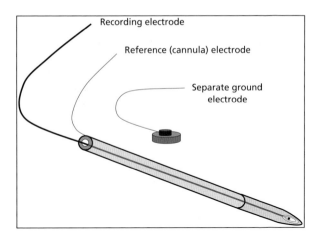

Figure 5.4
Bipolar concentric
needle.

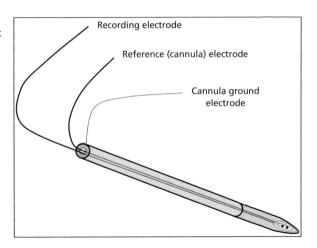

Bipolar Needle

The cannula of the bipolar needle contains two fine stainless steel or platinum wires (Fig. 5.4). This electrode is larger in diameter than the standard coaxial concentric needle. It registers the potential electrical difference between the two inside wires while the cannula serves as the ground. The bipolar needle detects potentials from a much smaller area than the standard coaxial concentric needle. This needle is also slightly more uncomfortable than a monopolar needle because of its increased diameter. This electrode is used primarily for research, not in routine clinical studies.

Single-fiber Needle

Single-fiber needles may wire exposed along the shaft serving as the leading edge to record from individual muscle fibers rather than motor units. These electrodes are used to assess neuromuscular junction transmission and fiber density, topics that are beyond the scope of this text.

Planning the Examination

It is important to plan out which muscles you will test before you begin. This plan may change, as you proceed, depending on the results of the muscles being tested. If you think the patient will only be able to tolerate a limited number of muscles, start with the ones that will contribute the most to your diagnosis. The test is uncomfortable, and many people are afraid of needles. Therefore, try to test as few muscles as possible without sacrificing the quality of the examination.

 ## Starting the Test

The EMG examination can be divided into four components:

- insertional activity
- examination of muscle at rest
- analyzing the motor unit
- recruitment.

Prior to evaluating insertional activity and examination of the muscle at rest it is important to make sure that the low frequency filter is set at 10–30 Hz and the high frequency filter is set at 10,000–20,000 Hz (10–20 kHz), the amplifier sensitivity is set at 50–100 microvolts per division and the sweep speed is usually set at 10 msec per division. The needle should be inserted into the muscle quickly and deliberately. Tensing the skin will allow quicker needle insertion and less discomfort to the patient.

For the first two components of the examination, insertional activity and examination of the resting muscle, the needle electrode is directed through the muscle in four quadrants. Each of these quadrants can be examined at three or four different depths, allowing 12 to 16 discrete areas of muscle to be examined electrically. The EMG has been likened to an 'electrical biopsy' and as with any biopsy the more areas examined the lower the chance of false negatives.

Insertional Activity

Healthy muscle at rest is electrically silent as soon as needle movement stops, as long as the endplate region is avoided. During this portion of the examination, the muscle being tested should be at rest. The best way to electrically silence the muscle (if the patient cannot relax the muscle) is to tell the patient to contract the antagonist muscle. For example, if you put a needle in the biceps muscle, and the patient's elbow is bent, motor units in the biceps muscle are probably firing. Telling the patient to straighten the elbow will activate motor units in the triceps muscle (and inactivate motor units in the biceps muscle). Since it is difficult to activate both the agonist and antagonist muscles at the same time, the agonist muscle usually will relax. (Remember that the biceps muscle is also a supinator. Therefore, pronating the arm is also important in order to put the biceps muscle at rest. Here again, a working knowledge of where muscles are, what they do, and what nerves innervate them is essential.)

If the needle is properly placed in the muscle you are testing you will hear and see brief electrical activity associated with the needle movement. This is called *insertional activity*. The sound associated with this needle movement has been described as 'crisp' and is temporally related to the high-frequency positive and negative spikes that are easily visualized on the monitor. This should be done in four different quadrants and at four different depths. To reposition the needle pull it back carefully to the plane where the muscle and fascia transition (with practice you will soon be able to 'feel' when you leave the muscle) and then insert at a new angle. Try not to pull back too far or you will pull the needle all the way out and have to restick the needle into the patient.

Normal insertional activity typically only lasts a few hundred milliseconds, just barely longer than the needle movement itself. It is thought to be generated by the needle tip physically depolarizing the muscle fibers as it pierces and/or displaces them.

Decreased insertional activity occurs when the needle is inserted into an *atrophied* muscle. The sensation of inserting the needle has been described as putting a needle into sand. Remember that the initial sound and electromyographic recording of needle insertion into muscle is actually the muscle fiber being injured by needle movement. With muscle atrophy, there will be decreased response to needle insertion, as there is less muscle tissue. Caution should be used in interpretation, especially without clinically visible muscle wasting, to make sure that the needle was indeed in muscle and not other tissue such as adipose or connective tissue.

Increased insertional activity may occur when there is muscle pathology and is evidenced by the presence of positive sharp waves and sometimes fibrillation potentials that are apparent only on insertion and *do not persist*. Increased insertional activity may precede actual denervation. On insertion, any electrical activity that lasts longer than 300 milliseconds is considered increased. These determinations require a subjective assessment based on the experience of the electromyographer (Fig. 5.5).

Examination of the Muscle at Rest

Once the needle is inserted into the muscle, pause several seconds to assess for spontaneous activity. Normal muscles should be electrically silent after needle insertion. For this portion of the test, the muscle should still be at rest.

Spontaneous Activity

Spontaneous activity is typically abnormal and occurs in the presence of pathology. Normal muscle has a resting membrane potential of –80 mv relative to the extracellular

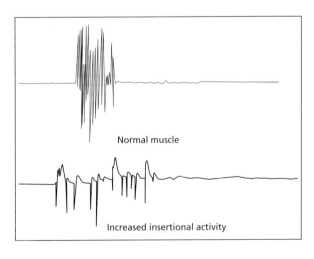

Figure 5.5 (Top) Normal insertional activity. (Bottom) Increased insertional activity.

Normal muscle

Increased insertional activity

fluids. After injury or denervation, the membrane potential becomes more positive due to an influx of Na^+ into the damaged cell membrane. The muscle cell tends to become less negative and therefore closer to the potential needed for the generation of spontaneous action potentials. This occurs when the cell resting membrane potential reaches –60 mv.

The term 'denervation potentials' is a misnomer and should not be used to describe spontaneous activity. Spontaneous activity is a more appropriate term. Irritation can be brought about by many factors other than nerve injury, such as metabolic and inflammatory muscle disease, and local muscle trauma. Either the muscle or the nerve may generate spontaneous activity (Table 5.1).

Positive sharp waves (PSW), fibrillations, complex repetitive discharges and myotonic discharges are examples of abnormal spontaneous potentials that are generated at the level of the muscle fiber. Abnormal findings, due to a dysfunction of the neural input to the muscle, can lead to the development of *myokymic* discharges as well as *cramps, neuromyotonic discharges, tremors, multiples and fasciculations*. The more common types of spontaneous activity will be described below. Because of their small amplitude, the gain on the EMG machine must be set to 50–100 microvolts for the potentials to be visualized.

Positive sharp waves (PSWs) are muscle fiber action potentials that can be recorded from a muscle with impaired muscle innervation or from an injured portion of a muscle. PSWs consist of a primary positive (downward) deflection from the baseline (positive wave), followed by a return to the baseline. These waves are either monophasic or biphasic in morphology (Fig. 5.6). They tend to fire regularly at a rate of 0.5 to 15 Hz, however, they also may have irregular firing patterns. Amplitudes tend to vary between 20 to 1000 microvolts with durations of 10–30 ms. PSWs sound like dull thuds, and tend to appear earlier than fibrillation potentials after muscle is deprived of its nerve supply.

Fibrillation potentials (fibs) are the spontaneous action potentials of single muscle fibers that are firing autonomously. This can occur in the presence of impaired innervation. This process repeats on a time interval dependent upon the repolarization-to-threshold turnaround time. These potentials usually fire in a regular pattern at rates of 0.5–15 Hz, although they may fire irregularly early after denervation. The fibrillation potentials are usually triphasic in morphology and range from 20 to 1000 microvolts in size (Fig. 5.7). They sound like raindrops hitting a tin roof. Fibrillation potentials and

Table 5.1 Spontaneous activity generated by muscle or nerve

Spontaneous activity generated by the muscle – fibrillation potentials (fibs) – positive sharp wave (PSW) – myotonic discharges – complex repetitive discharges
Spontaneous activity generated by the nerve – myokymic discharges – cramps – neuromyotonic discharges – tremors – multiples (multiple motor unit potentials, i.e. doublets or triplets) – *fasciculations
*Fasciculations can be considered muscle or nerve generated.

Figure 5.6
Positive sharp
wave.

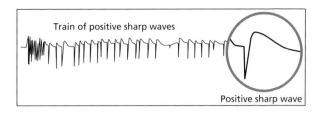

Positive sharp wave

Figure 5.7
Fibrillation.

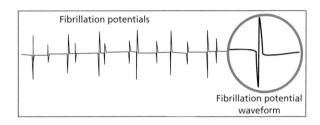

Table 5.2 Conditions associated with positive sharp waves and fibrillation potential

Chronic muscle disorders
- inflammatory myopathies
- muscular dystrophies
- inclusion body myositis
- congenital myopathies
- rhabdomyolysis
- muscle trauma
- trichinosis

Neurogenic disorders
- radiculopathy
- axonal peripheral neuropathy
- plexopathies
- entrapment neuropathies
- motor neuron disease
- mononeuropathies

PSWs may be recorded from both neurogenic and myopathic disease states and when seen on EMG essentially signifies the same thing – spontaneous discharge of the muscle fibers most often due to impaired innervation of the muscle being tested (Table 5.2).

Spontaneous fibs and PSWs are usually reported on a scale of zero to four. Zero means that no fibs or PSWs are present. The rest of the grading is subjective. As a general rule, if one PSW or fib is seen per screen (using a sweep of 10 milliseconds per division) the score is +1. In this situation, the fibs or PSWs may not be present in every area of the muscle. If spontaneous potentials are present in more areas of the muscle or are more numerous, the score is +2. If fibs and PSWs essentially fill the screen, they are graded as +4.

Fibs and PSWs usually indicate a process of acute or ongoing impaired innervation. These spontaneous potentials however, may not be seen on EMG testing until three weeks or more after an injury. See Chapter 6 for further details on timing of EMG findings after nerve injury.

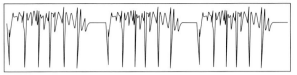

Figure 5.8
Complex
repetitive
discharge.

Table 5.3 Conditions associated with complex repetitive discharges

Chronic muscle disorders
– myopathies
– inflammatory
– limb-girdle dystrophy
– myxedema
– Schwartz–Jampel syndrome

Neurogenic disorders
– chronic neuropathies or radiculopathies
– poliomyelitis
– spinal muscular atrophy
– motor neuron disease
– hereditary neuropathies

Complex repetitive discharges (CRD) are groups of spontaneously firing action potentials. The etiology of the CRD is a local muscular 'arrhythmia' with an affected area of muscle electrically stimulating adjacent muscle fibers and therefore perpetuating the rhythm. They appear as runs of simple or complex spike patterns that repeat in a regular pattern. They have a frequency of 10–100 Hz. The amplitudes of the responses are between 50 and 500 microvolts. These potentials start and stop abruptly (Fig. 5.8). They have a uniform frequency, and sound like a motorboat that misfires occasionally. These potentials are seen in both neurogenic and myopathic disorders (Table 5.3). They tend to be seen in more longstanding disorders and are suggestive that the injury is greater than six months old.

Myotonic discharges are the action potentials of muscle fibers firing in a prolonged fashion after activation. Clinically this is seen as delayed relaxation of a muscle after a forceful contraction. This may also be seen after striking a muscle belly with a reflex hammer, as in percussion myotonia. Myotonic discharges have two potential forms. The wave may either have PSW morphology or a pattern of biphasic or triphasic potentials. These potentials tend to fire at a variable rate with a waxing and waning appearance. The frequency varies between 20 to 100Hz (Fig. 5.9). This variation in frequency gives the discharge its characteristic 'dive bomber' sound. Myotonic discharges are found in the following conditions: myotonic dystrophy, myotonia congenita, paramyotonia, hyperkalemic periodic paralysis, polymyositis, acid maltase deficiency and chronic radiculopathy and neuropathies.

Myokymic discharges are groups of spontaneous motor unit potentials that have a regular firing pattern and rhythm. They are seen in two forms. In the continuous form they are seen as single or paired discharges of motor unit potentials that fire at rates of 5–10 Hz. In the discontinuous form they are seen as bursts of motor potentials, which repeat at 0.1–10 Hz. This form of the myokymic response sounds like soldiers marching (Fig. 5.10). Myokymic responses may be seen in facial muscles in Bell's palsy, multiple sclerosis, and polyradiculopathy. They are also seen in limb muscles in chronic nerve

Figure 5.9
Myotonic
discharges.

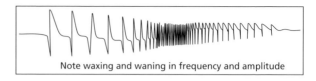

Note waxing and waning in frequency and amplitude

Figure 5.10
Myokymic
discharges.

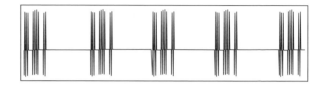

lesions and in radiation plexopathy. The term myokymia is used clinically to describe a 'worm-like' quivering of the muscle. However, this clinical finding is usually associated with neuromyotonic, rather than myokymic discharges, on EMG.

Endplate Region

Healthy muscle should have no *spontaneous activity*, unless the needle is in the endplate region of a muscle fiber (where the nerve enters the muscle). If the needle is in the endplate region, it should be repositioned, as you are not likely to ascertain anything about a muscle from this location and it can be quite painful for the patient. There are three things to look for that may tell you the needle is in the endplate region:

1. *MEPPs* (miniature endplate potentials)
2. *Endplate spikes*
3. *Pain* (the patient may feel a dull ache or increased pain relative to other positions).

MEPPs are believed to represent the spontaneous release of acetylcholine (Ach) at the presynaptic terminal. When Ach attaches to the receptors there is subsequent activation of the sodium and potassium channels of the muscle, which in turn creates a small current.

Endplate spikes are believed to be single muscle fiber depolarizations. A needle may cause sufficient irritation to the presynaptic nerve terminal to release a large amount of Ach. This may subsequently produce a threshold adequate for depolarization.

Endplate spikes and MEPPs do not necessarily have to be found together. *MEPPs* are of short duration (1–2 milliseconds), fire with irregular activity every few seconds or so, are small in size (10–20 microvolts), and have monophasic negative (upward) waveforms (Fig. 5.11). *Endplate spikes* are typically biphasic with an initial negative deflection, of intermediate amplitude (about 100–200 microvolts), and have longer duration than MEPPs (3–5 milliseconds). Like MEPPs, they fire irregularly. The endplates should be avoided because of patient discomfort and possible interpretation errors. (Positive waves in the endplate do not indicate denervation, and can be a normal finding.) To move away from the endplate, advance the needle slightly and firmly. Now the muscle should be electrically quiet and the patient more comfortable.

Analyzing the Motor Unit

Once the muscle has been assessed for insertional activity and activity at rest, the motor unit itself should be analyzed. During this portion of the needle test, the patient is asked

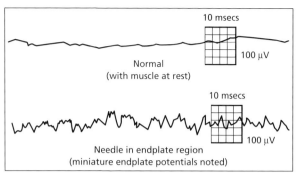

Figure 5.11
Miniature
endplate
potential (MEPP).

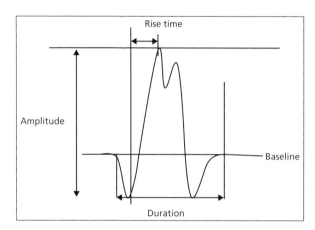

Figure 5.12
MUAP
components.

to *minimally* contract the muscle. Too often, electromyographers tell the patient to maximally contract the muscle. If the muscle is fully contracted, it is almost impossible to isolate and therefore analyze individual motor units.

When analyzing motor units, the sweep speed should be set at 10 msec/division and the gain should be 200–500 microvolts per division. Most assessments of motor unit morphology can be made more accurately by freezing the screen or by using a trigger and delay line. Trigger and delay lines are available on most EMG machines by pressing a button. This is necessary for a detailed analysis of motor units. The trigger is set to record a tracing when a certain amplitude threshold is reached. When a potential exceeds the trigger threshold, that potential is displayed on the screen. That potential remains on the screen until the next potential reaches threshold. Then the new potential replaces the previous potential. This allows the electromyographer to 'freeze' a MUAP above certain amplitude and analyze it.

At low levels of contraction (when few motor units are firing), slight movements of the needle can 'tune in' the desired potential. At this point, the same potential will be constantly replaced in the same location on the screen. The delay line determines the position of the potential on the screen. Thus, the placement of the delay line determines how much time before and after the potential being examined is being displayed. The 'strobe' effect of potentials being locked into the same position allows detailed analysis of all components of motor unit morphology including amplitude, duration and number of phases as well as stability. Subtle changes can become apparent.

In addition, satellite potentials, separated from the main motor unit action potential by an isoelectric interval, fire in a time-locked relationship to the main action potential. These potentials usually follow, but may precede, the main action potential in the same location and therefore will become apparent. These will likely only be evident in this manner, as without a trigger and delay function they may appear as different motor units. The trigger and delay function is an extremely valuable tool in performing motor unit analysis.

Components of the Motor Unit

Analysis of the motor unit morphology should include the following parameters: 1. amplitude, 2. rise time, 3. duration and 4. phases. Figure 5.12 depicts the various components of the MUAP morphology.

Amplitude

In a healthy motor unit, all of the muscle fibers discharge in near synchrony. Muscle fibers located near the tip of the electrode make the greatest contribution to the amplitude of the motor unit potential. Their contribution to the amplitude decreases significantly as the distance from the needle tip increases. Therefore the *same* motor unit can give rise to potentials of *different* amplitude and appearance at different recording sites.

MUAP amplitude is measured from the most positive to the most negative peak, and reflects fiber density. Amplitude of the motor units may be *normal, increased or decreased*. With a concentric needle, amplitude ranges from several hundred microvolts to a few millivolts. Amplitudes are larger with a monopolar needle because the monopolar needle picks up electrical activity from a full 360-degree field around the needle. Increased amplitude of motor units can be seen with reinnervation, as is seen with neuropathic injuries after a period of months. Decreased amplitude may be seen in myopathies.

Rise Time

Rise time is the time lag from the peak of the initial positive deflection to the subsequent negative upward peak. This helps estimate the distance between the recording tip and discharging motor unit. The more vertical the waveform, the shorter (quicker) the rise time. A distant motor unit has longer rise time because the resistance and capacitance of the intervening tissue act as a high frequency filter. A unit accepted for qualitative measurement should produce a sharp sound, while a distant unit will produce a dull sound indicating the need to reposition the needle electrode closer to the source. An acceptable rise time is 0.5 milliseconds or less.

Duration

Duration is measured from the initial departure from baseline to the final return to the baseline. Normal duration is about 5–15 milliseconds. It indicates the degree of synchrony of firing among all individual muscle fibers with variable length, conduction velocity and membrane excitability. A slight shift in the needle position influences the duration much less than the amplitude.

When all the fibers of a motor unit fire in relative synchrony, the duration will be short. If there is asynchrony of firing (e.g., with reinnervation) the duration will be longer. Increased duration is seen in neuropathic processes, while decreased duration is seen in myopathic disorders. Duration is decreased in myopathies because fewer muscle fibers contribute to the motor unit.

Phases

A phase is the portion of the waveform between the successive crossings of the baseline. The number of phases, determined by counting negative and positive peaks, equals the number of baseline crossing plus one. Normally, motor unit potentials have four or fewer phases. Polyphasic motor units (more than four phases) suggest desynchronized discharge or drop-off of individual fibers. Normal muscles may have about 10% polyphasic MUAPs using a concentric needle and 25% polyphasic MUAPs when using a monopolar needle. If more than approximately 20% of the motor units analyzed with a concentric needle or 40% with a monopolar needle consist of five or more phases, the motor units of that muscle are considered polyphasic. Motor unit duration is a better measure of pathology than polyphasicity.

Remember that the spatial relationship between the needle and the muscle fibers plays an important role in the shape of the waveform, so any slight repositioning of the electrode can change the morphology of the motor unit.

Recruitment

Recruitment is an often misunderstood and misused term. Recruitment refers to the *orderly addition of motor units* so as to *increase the force of a contraction.* A contraction becomes stronger in two ways: the firing motor units *increase their rate of firing* and *additional motor units commence firing.*

The settings on the machine for evaluating recruitment should be a sweep of 10 milliseconds per division and a gain of 200–500 microvolts per division. Recruitment analysis should begin with the patient being told to think about contracting the muscle being analyzed. Observe for the firing of a single MUAP. It usually begins to fire at 2–3 Hz in an *irregular* pattern.

Normally the motor unit will fire in a *regular* pattern at about 5Hz. At around 10 Hz another MUAP will be recruited to fire. The new motor unit (MU) will initially fire at about 5 Hz. The normal firing rate of most motor units, before additional units are recruited, is 10 Hz. To calculate the firing rate of the MU, note how many times a MU with an identical morphology repeats across a screen set at 100 msec/screen (sweep speed of 10 msec/division). Multiply that number by ten to get the motor unit firing per 1000 msec or one second. Remember that Hz indicates cycles per second. In neuropathic processes, some motor units will be unavailable to fire (see Fig. 5.13). A MU that is able to fire will try to 'make up' for the inability of other units to fire by firing at a higher frequency. Therefore, the motor unit will have an increased firing frequency before another motor unit is recruited, which is referred to as decreased recruitment. In decreased recruitment, there are fewer motor units firing at higher frequency. Recruitment ratio is another term used to describe the firing rate of a motor unit. This ratio is the rate of firing of the most rapidly firing motor unit (in Hz) divided by the number of units firing. A recruitment ratio of over 8 is considered abnormal and suggests a neurogenic process.

Neuropathic recruitment, also called neurogenic recruitment, can be seen in neuropathies, radiculopathies, motor neuron disease and nerve trauma. Few motor units fire at an increased rate, or firing frequency (Fig. 5.13). The firing rates of these MUAPs are greater than 20 Hz (20 cycles per second) and may increase to over 30 Hz or more. Pathologic states can tell us much about physiology. In severe neuropathic lesions, when there are few functional motor units, we can see motor units firing at 30 Hz before a second motor unit in that area is recruited. This indicates that weakness is not due to pain or poor effort, but due to physiologic factors. Functional motor units are simply not

Figure 5.13
Schematic of normal, neuropathic and myopathic processes.

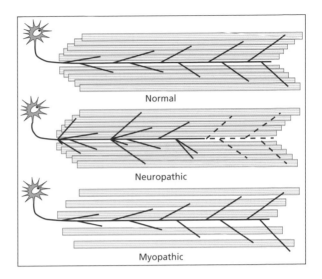

available. If only a few motor units are firing but they are firing at a normal rate, recruitment is normal. The decreased activation of the muscle may be due to either decreased effort or a central nervous system lesion.

The term 'increased recruitment' or 'early recruitment' is sometimes used to describe a myopathic process. In myopathic recruitment, a large number of motor units are 'recruited' for a minimal contraction. In myopathies, the individual muscle fiber contribution to each motor unit is reduced (see Fig. 5.13). Since myopathic motor units cannot increase their force output, they quickly recruit additional motor units to increase the force of a contraction. If referring to the recruitment ratio, there will be a decreased rate of firing (numerator) per number of motor units recruited (denominator). Recruitment ratios below 3 suggest a myopathic process.

Myopathic MUAPs tend to have an *early* recruitment of *short* duration *low* amplitude MUAPs firing at increased rates (Fig. 5.14). In a myopathy it is difficult to obtain only one or two motor units per screen at minimal contraction. Polyphasicity and spontaneous potentials can be seen in both neuropathies and myopathies. Because these motor units have low amplitude, analysis cannot be done as easily with a trigger and delay or capture function but must be done with a constant sweep.

In EMG evaluation of MUAP recruitment, it is important to realize that we are primarily evaluating Type I motor units because they recruit first. By the time the Type II fibers recruit, the baseline will be obscured by Type I potentials. This is problematic in those myopathies that involve predominately Type II fibers, such as steroid myopathies, since only the Type I fibers are evaluated. In steroid myopathies, even though the patient has a myopathy clinically and on biopsy, the EMG may be normal.

 ## Summary

EMG evaluation requires patience and effort on the part of both the electromyographer and the patient. The amount of information obtained from the test is dependent upon appropriate planning and selection of the muscles as well as experience in waveform recognition. Table 5.4 reviews the common muscles tested during the needle portion of the

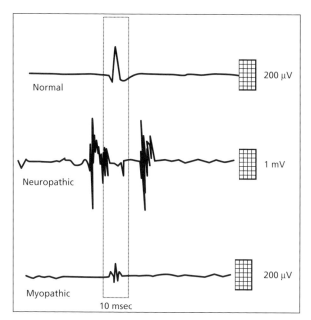

Figure 5.14
Normal, neuropathic and myopathic recruitment.

examination, as well as the muscle's innervation, location and needle placement. This will help you plan out which muscles to test as well as ensure proper needle placement. This is a relatively comprehensive list and it is rare that most or even many of these muscles will be necessary in an individual study. The choice of muscles examined should be dictated by the clinical circumstances.

Many muscles are very close together (in the forearm for example), and due to individual differences in size (and less often to differences in anatomy), as well as depth of needle insertion, the needle may not always be in the desired muscle. A test maneuver may be necessary to confirm needle placement. Activating the muscle tests placement. If the needle is in the muscle being activated, large crisp motor units will be seen and heard. Videotapes that can be a valuable tool in waveform recognition are available from the American Association of Electrodiagnostic Medicine (AAEM).

Table 5.4 Common muscles – innervation, location and needle placement

Muscle	Nerve	Cord	Division	Trunk	C4	C5
Sternoclei-domastoid (see Fig. A2.1)	Spinal Accessory Nerve					
Trapezius (see Fig. A2.2)	Spinal Accessory Nerve	CN XI, C3				
Rhomboid Major (see Fig. A2.3)	Dorsal Scapular Nerve	N/A	N/A	N/A		C5
Rhomboid Minor (see Fig. A2.3)	Dorsal Scapular Nerve	N/A	N/A	N/A		C5
Levator Scapulae (see Fig. A2.4)	Dorsal Scapular Nerve	N/A	N/A	N/A	C3, C4	C5
Supraspinatus (see Fig. A2.5)	Suprascapular Nerve	N/A	N/A	Upper Trunk		C5

C6	C7	C8	T1	Needle Insertion	Origin	Insertion	Action
				At the midpoint between the mastoid process and the sternal origin; enter the muscle obliquely, and direct the needle parallel to the muscle fibers	The sternal head arises from the upper part of the manubrium sterni. The clavicular head arises from the medial third of the clavicle	The lateral surface of the mastoid process	Rotates the head
				At the angle of the neck and shoulder or midway between the spine of the scapula and the spinous processes at the same level	External occipital protuberance, superior nuchal line, ligamentum nuchae, spines of C7–T12	Spine of scapula, acromion, lateral third of clavicle	Adducts, rotates, elevates, and depresses scapula
				At the midpoint of the medial scapular border, midway between the scapular spine and the inferior angle beneath the trapezius	Spines of T2–T5	Medial border of scapula	Adducts scapula
				At the point just medially to medial border of the scapular spine beneath the trapezius	Spines of C7–T1	Root of spine of scapula	Adducts scapula
				At the posteromedial border of the scapula, between the superior angle and the spine of the scapula beneath the trapezius	The transverse processes of the upper four cervical vertebrae	The postero-medial border of the scapula, between the superior angle and the spine of the scapula	Elevates the scapula
C6				At the supraspinous fossa just above the spine of the scapula beneath the trapezius	Supraspinous fossa of scapula	Superior facet of greater tubercle of humerus	Abducts arm

Table 5.4 Common muscles – innervation, location and needle placement (*cont'd*)

Muscle	Nerve	Cord	Division	Trunk	C4	C5
Infraspinatus (see Fig. A2.6)	Suprascapular Nerve	N/A	N/A	Upper Trunk		C5
Subscapularis	Upper and Lower Subscapular Nerve	Posterior Cord	Posterior Division	Upper Trunk		C5
Teres Major (see Fig. A2.7)	Lower Subscapular Nerve	Posterior Cord	Posterior Division	Upper Trunk and Middle Trunk		C5
Deltoid (see Fig. A2.8)	Axillary Nerve	Posterior Cord	Posterior Division	Upper Trunk		C5
Teres Minor (see Fig. A2.9)	Axillary Nerve	Posterior Cord	Posterior Division	Upper Trunk		C5
Coracobrachialis (see Fig. A2.10)	Musculocutaneous Nerve	Lateral Cord	Anterior Division	Upper and Middle Trunk		C5
Biceps Brachii (see Fig. A2.11)	Musculocutaneous Nerve	Lateral Cord	Anterior Division	Upper Trunk		C5
Brachialis (see Fig. A2.12)	Musculocutaneous Nerve	Lateral Cord	Anterior Division	Upper Trunk		C5
Latissimus Dorsi (see Fig. A2.13)	Thoracodorsal Nerve	Posterior Cord	Posterior Division	Upper, Middle and Lower Trunk		

C6	C7	C8	T1	Needle Insertion	Origin	Insertion	Action
C6				At the midpoint of infraspinous fossa beneath the trapezius	Infraspinous fossa	Middle facet of greater tubercle of humerus	Externally rotates arm
C6					Subscapular fossa	Lesser tubercle of humerus	Internally rotates arm
C6	C7			Along the lateral lower border of the scapula (lateral and rostral to the inferior angle) beneath the trapezius	Dorsal surface of inferior angle of scapula	Medial lip of inter-tubercular groove of humerus	Internally adducts and rotates arm
C6				5 cm beneath the lateral border of the acromion	Lateral third of clavicle, acromion, and spine of scapula	Deltoid tuberosity of humerus	Abducts, flexes, extends, and internally and externally rotates arm
C6				Immediately lateral to the middle third of the lateral border of the scapula	Upper portion of lateral border of scapula	Lower facet of greater tubercle of humerus	Externally rotates arm
C6	C7			5–9 cm distal to the coracoid process along the volar aspect of the arm	Coracoid process	Middle third of medial surface of humerus	Flexes and adducts arm
C6				At the midarm anteriorly, into bulk of the muscle	Long head, supraglenoid tubercle; short head, coracoid process	Radial tuberosity of radius	Flexes and supinates forearm; assists in flexion of arm at shoulder
C6				5 cm proximal to the elbow crease just lateral to and under the biceps	Lower anterior surface of humerus	Coronoid process of ulna and ulnar tuberosity	Flexes forearm at elbow
C6	C7	C8		Along the posterior axillary fold directly lateral to the inferior angle of the scapula	Spines of T7–T12 thoracolumbar fascia, iliac crest, ribs 9–12	Floor of bicipital groove of humerus	Adducts, extends, and internally rotates arm

Table 5.4 Common muscles – innervation, location and needle placement (*cont'd*)

Muscle	Nerve	Cord	Division	Trunk	C4	C5
Serratus Anterior (see Fig. A2.14)	Long Thoracic Nerve	Anterior Rami				C5
Triceps (see Fig. A2.15)	Radial Nerve	Posterior Cord	Posterior Division	Upper, Middle and Lower Trunk		
Anconeus (see Fig. A2.16)	Radial Nerve	Posterior Cord	Posterior Division	Upper, Middle and Lower Trunk		
Brachioradialis (see Fig. A2.17)	Radial Nerve	Posterior Cord	Posterior Division	Upper Trunk		C5
Extensor carpi radialis (see Fig. A2.18)	Radial Nerve	Posterior Cord	Posterior Division	Upper and Middle Trunk		
Supinator (see Fig. A2.19)	Posterior Interosseous Nerve (Radial Nerve)	Posterior Cord	Posterior Division	Upper Trunk		C5
Extensor Carpi Ulnaris (see Fig. A2.20)	Posterior Interosseous Nerve (Radial Nerve)	Posterior Cord	Posterior Division	Middle and Lower Trunk		

C6	C7	C8	T1	Needle Insertion	Origin	Insertion	Action
C6	C7			Along the midaxillary line directly over the rib, anterior to the bulk of the latissimus dorsi but, in a woman, posterior to breast tissue	At the outer surfaces and superior borders of the upper eight or nine ribs	The medial border of the scapula, from the superior angle to the costal surface of the inferior angle	Protracts scapula; assists upward rotation of scapula
C6	C7	C8		At the midarm level posterior to the lateral aspect of the shaft of the humerus	Long head, infraglenoid tubercle; lateral head, superior to radial groove of humerus; medial head, inferior to radial groove	Posterior surface of olecranon process of ulna	Extends the elbow
C6	C7	C8		2.5–3.75 cm distal to the olecranon along the radial border of the ulna	Lateral epicondyle of humerus	Olecranon and upper posterior surface of ulna	Extends forearm
C6				2–3 cm lateral to the biceps tendon	Lateral supracondylar ridge of humerus	Base of radial styloid process	Flexes forearm
C6	C7			At the upper forearm 5–7.5 cm distal to the lateral epicondyle along a line connecting the epicondyle and second metacarpal bone	Lower third of the lateral supracondylar ridge of the humerus	Radial surface of the base of the second and third metacarpal bone	Extends (dorsi-flexion) and radially abducts hand at wrist
C6				With the forearm pronated, insert the needle 3–5 cm distal to the lateral epicondyle, toward the shaft of the radius	Lateral epicondyle, radial collateral and annular ligaments	Lateral side of upper part of radius	Supinates forearm
	C7	C8		With the forearm pronated, at the mid to upper forearm just radial to the lateral margin of the shaft of the ulna	The common extensor tendon from the lateral epicondyle of the humerus	At the ulnar side of the base of the fifth metacarpal bone	Extends (dorsi-flexion) and ulnarly deviates hand at wrist

Table 5.4 Common muscles – innervation, location and needle placement (*cont'd*)

Muscle	Nerve	Cord	Division	Trunk	C4	C5
Extensor Digitorum (see Fig. A2.21)	Posterior Interosseous Nerve (Radial Nerve)	Posterior Cord	Posterior Division	Middle and Lower Trunk		
Extensor Digiti Minimi (see Fig. A2.22)	Posterior Interosseous Nerve (Radial Nerve)	Posterior Cord	Posterior Division	Middle and Lower Trunk		
Abductor Pollicis Longus (see Fig. A2.23)	Posterior Interosseous Nerve (Radial Nerve)	Posterior Cord	Posterior Division	Middle and Lower Trunk		
Extensor Pollicis Longus (see Fig. A2.24)	Posterior Interosseous Nerve (Radial Nerve)	Posterior Cord	Posterior Division	Middle and Lower Trunk		
Extensor Pollicis Brevis (see Fig. A2.25)	Posterior Interosseous Nerve (Radial Nerve)	Posterior Cord	Posterior Division	Middle and Lower Trunk		
Extensor Indicis (see Fig. A2.26)	Posterior Interosseous Nerve (Radial Nerve)	Posterior Cord	Posterior Division	Middle and Lower Trunk		
Pronator Teres (see Fig. A2.27)	Median Nerve	Lateral Cord	Anterior Division	Upper and Middle Trunk		
Flexor Carpi Radialis (see Fig. A2.28)	Median Nerve	Lateral Cord	Anterior Division	Upper and Middle Trunk		

C6	C7	C8	T1	Needle Insertion	Origin	Insertion	Action
	C7	C8		With the forearm pronated, at mid-forearm, midway between the ulna and radius	Common extensor tendon from the lateral epicondyle of the humerus	The dorsal surface of all phalanges of digits 2 through 4	Extends phalanges in digits 2 through 4
	C7	C8		With the forearm pronated, at mid-forearm mid-way between the ulna and radius	Common extensor tendon and interosseous membrane	Extensor expansion, base of middle and distal phalanges	Extends little finger
	C7	C8		With the forearm pronated, at the mid-forearm along the shaft of the radius	Interosseous membrane, middle third of posterior surfaces of radius and ulna	Lateral surface of base of first metacarpal	Abducts thumb radially
	C7	C8		With the forearm pronated, at the mid-forearm along the radial border of the ulna	Interosseous membrane and middle third of posterior surface of ulna	Base of distal phalanx of thumb	Extends all parts of thumb but specifically extension of distal phalanx; assists adduction of thumb
	C7	C8		4–6 cm proximal to the wrist over the ulnar aspect of the radius	Interosseous membrane and posterior surface of middle third radius	Base of proximal phalanx of thumb	Extends proximal phalanx of thumb
	C7	C8		5–7 cm proximal to the ulnar styloid just radial to the shaft of the ulna	Posterior surface of ulna and interosseous membrane	Extensor expansion of index finger	Extends index finger
C6	C7			With the arm supinated, at 2–3 cm distal and 1 cm medial to the biceps tendon	Medial epicondyle and coronoid process of ulna	Middle of lateral side of radius	Pronates forearm
C6	C7			With the arm supinated, at the volar surface of the forearm, 7–9 cm distal to the medial epicondyle along a line directed toward the muscle tendon at the wrist	Medial epicondyle of the humerus	Volar surface of the base of the second metacarpal	Flexes hand at wrist (palmar flexion); assists in radial abduction of hand

Table 5.4 Common muscles – innervation, location and needle placement (*cont'd*)

Muscle	Nerve	Cord	Division	Trunk	C4	C5
Palmaris Longus (see Fig. A2.29)	Median Nerve	Lateral and Medial Cord	Anterior Division	Middle Trunk and Lower Trunk		
Flexor Digitorum Superficialis (see Fig. A2.30)	Median Nerve	Lateral and Medial Cord	Anterior Division	Middle Trunk and Lower Trunk		
Flexor Digitorum Profundus (see Fig. A2.31)	Anterior Interosseous Nerve (Median Nerve) and Ulnar Nerve	Lateral and Medial Cord	Anterior Division	Middle Trunk and Lower Trunk		
Flexor Pollicis Longus (see Fig. A2.32)	Anterior Interosseous Nerve (Median Nerve)	Lateral and Medial Cord	Anterior Division	Middle Trunk and Lower Trunk		
Pronator Quadratus (see Fig. A2.27)	Anterior Interosseous Nerve (Median Nerve)	Lateral and Medial Cord	Anterior Division	Middle Trunk and Lower Trunk		
Abductor Pollicis Brevis (see Fig. A2.33)	Median Nerve	Medial Cord	Anterior Division	Lower Trunk		

C6	C7	C8	T1	Needle Insertion	Origin	Insertion	Action
	C7	C8	T1	With the arm supinated at the volar surface of the forearm 6–8 cm distal to the medial epicondyle along a line directed toward the muscle tendon at the wrist	Medial epicondyle of humerus	Flexor retinaculum, palmar aponeurosis	Flexes hand at wrist
	C7	C8	T1	With the arm supinated, at the volar surface of the forearm approximately 7–9 cm distal to the biceps tendon (mid forearm) and 2–3 cm medial to the ventral midline	Medial epicondyle of the humerus by the common tendon, coronoid process of ulna, and oblique line of the radius	The sides of the second phalanges of digits 2 through 5	Flexes the proximal interphalangeal joints
	C7	C8	T1	With the arm supinated, at 5–7.5 cm distal to the olecranon process and 1–1.5 cm medial to the shaft of the ulna	Anteromedial surface of ulna, interosseous membrane	Bases of distal phalanges of fingers	Flexes distal phalanges of fingers; assists in flexion of hand at wrist
	C7	C8	T1	With the arm supinated, 5–7.5 cm proximal to the radial styloid and 0.1 cm lateral to the radial artery	Anterior surface of radius, interosseous membrane, and coronoid process	Base of distal phalanx of thumb	Flexes thumb, particularly distal phalanx; assists in ulnar adduction of thumb
	C7	C8	T1	2.5 cm proximal to the ulnar styloid, midpoint between radial and ulna bone, deep to 2.5 cm to penetrate the interosseous membrane	The distal fourth of the volar surface of the ulna	The distal fourth of the lateral border and the volar surface of the radius	Pronates forearm
		C8	T1	Obliquely near the muscle origin along the muscle, midway along the shaft of the 1st metacarpal	Flexor retinaculum, scaphoid, and trapezium	Lateral side of base of proximal phalanx of thumb	Abducts thumb

Table 5.4 Common muscles – innervation, location and needle placement (*cont'd*)

Muscle	Nerve	Cord	Division	Trunk	C4	C5
Opponens Pollicis (see Fig. A2.34)	Median Nerve	Medial Cord	Anterior Division	Lower Trunk		
Flexor Pollicis Brevis (see Fig. A2.35)	Median Nerve: superficial head. Ulnar Nerve: deep head.	Medial Cord	Anterior Division	Lower Trunk		
Flexor Carpi Ulnaris (see Fig. A2.36)	Ulnar Nerve	Medial Cord	Anterior Division	Lower Trunk		
Abductor digiti minimi (see Fig. A2.37)	Ulnar Nerve	Medial Cord	Anterior Division	Lower Trunk		
Opponens digiti minimi (see Fig. A2.38)	Ulnar Nerve	Medial Cord	Anterior Division	Lower Trunk		

C6	C7	C8	T1	Needle Insertion	Origin	Insertion	Action
		C8	T1	Lateral to the APB, the most lateral part of the thenar eminence	Flexor retinaculum and trapezium	Lateral side of first metacarpal	Moves first metacarpal across palm and rotates it into opposition
		C8	T1	Superficial head: a depth of 0.5–1 cm at the midpoint of a line drawn between the metacarpo-phalangeal joint and the pisiform. Deep head: the same as that for the superficial head, but insert the needle to a depth of 1–2 cm	The superficial head originates in the flexor retinaculum and trapezium. The deep head originates in the ulnar aspect of the first metacarpal bone	The superficial head is inserted at the radial aspect of the base of the proximal phalanx of the thumb. The deep head is inserted at the ulnar aspect of the base of the proximal phalanx of the thumb	Flexes proximal phalanx of thumb; assists in opposition, ulnar adduction (entire muscle), and palmar abduction (superficial head) of thumb
		C8	T1	5–8 cm distal to the medial epicondyle along a line connecting the medial epicondyle and pisiform bone	Lateral epicondyle and posterior surface of ulna	Base of fifth metacarpal	Flexes and ulnarly deviates hand at wrist
		C8	T1	Insert the needle obliquely at the midpoint of the 5th metacarpal along the ulnar (medial) border of the hand	Pisiform and tendon of flexor carpi ulnaris	Pisiform and tendon of flexor carpi ulnaris	Abducts little finger
		C8	T1	The midpoint between the 5th metacar-pophalangeal joint (metacar-pophalangeal crease) and the pisiform (distal wrist crease), just radial to the abductor digiti minimi	Flexor retinaculum and hook of hamate	Medial side of fifth metacarpal	Opposes little finger

Table 5.4 Common muscles – innervation, location and needle placement (*cont'd*)

Muscle	Nerve	Cord	Division	Trunk	C4	C5
Flexor digiti minimi (see Fig. A2.39)	Ulnar Nerve	Medial Cord	Anterior Division	Lower Trunk		
Palmar Interosseous (see Fig. A2.40)	Ulnar Nerve	Medial Cord	Anterior Division	Lower Trunk		
First Dorsal Interosseous (see Fig. A2.41)	Ulnar Nerve	Medial Cord	Anterior Division	Lower Trunk		
Adductor Pollicis (see Fig. A2.42)	Ulnar Nerve	Medial Cord	Anterior Division	Lower Trunk		
Lumbricals (4) (see Fig. A2.43)	Median Nerve (two lateral) and Ulnar Nerve (two medial)	Medial Cord	Anterior Division	Lower Trunk		

C6	C7	C8	T1	Needle Insertion	Origin	Insertion	Action
		C8	T1	The midpoint between the fifth metacarpo-phalangeal joint (metacarpo-phalangeal crease) and the ulnar aspect of the pisiform (distal wrist crease), just radial to the opponens digiti minimi	The hook of the hamate and the flexor retinaculum	The ulnar side of the base of the proximal phalanx of the little finger	Flexes proximal phalanx of the fifth digit
		C8	T1	Just ulnar to the 2nd metacarpal bone or just radial to the 4th and 5th metacarpal bones, respectively on the palmer surface of the hand	Medial side of second metacarpal; lateral sides of fourth and fifth metacarpals	Bases of proximal phalanges in same sides as their origins; extensor expansion	Adducts fingers; flexes metacarpo-phalangeal joints; extends interpha-langeal joints.
		C8	T1	Obliquely just proximal to the 2nd metacarpo-phalangeal joint, and direct it rostrally along the muscle belly on the dorsum of the hand	The ulnar border of the first metacarpal bone (outer head) and the radial border of the second metacarpal bone (inner head)	The radial aspect of the base of the proximal phalanx of the index finger	Abducts the index finger (radial deviation)
		C8	T1	The first web space just anterior (volar) to the edge of the first dorsal interosseous and proximal to the first metacarpo-phalangeal joint on the palmar surface of the hand	Capitate and bases of second and third metacarpals (oblique head); palmar surface of third metacarpal (transverse head)	Medial side of base of proximal phalanx of the thumb	Adducts thumb
		C8	T1	Proximal to the metacarpopha-langeal joint and radial to the flexor tendon on the Palmar surface of the hand	Lateral side of tendons of flexor digitorum profundus	Lateral side of extensor expansion	Flexes metacarpo-phalangeal joints and extends inter-phalangeal joints

Table 5.4 Common muscles – innervation, location and needle placement (*cont'd*)

Muscle	Nerve	Cord	Division	Trunk	C4	C5
Pectoralis major (see Fig. A2.44)	Lateral and Medial Pectoral Nerves	Lateral Cord and Medial	Anterior Division	Upper, Middle, and Lower Trunk		C5
Pectoralis minor (see Fig. A2.44)	Medial Pectoral Nerve and Lateral/and Medial	Lateral Cord	Anterior Division	Upper, Middle, and Lower Trunk		C5

C6	C7	C8	T1	Needle Insertion	Origin	Insertion	Action
C6	C7	C8	T1	Medial to the anterior axillary fold over the bulk of the muscle	The clavicular part originates at the sternal half of the clavicle. The sternocostal part originates at the anterior surface of the sternum, the edge of the first six or seven ribs, and the aponeurosis of the external oblique muscle of the abdomen	The lateral lip of the inter-tubercular sulcus on the shaft of the humerus	Adducts and internally rotates arm. Clavicular portion: assists in flexion of arm
C6	C7	C8	T1	The midclavicular line overlying the third rib	The outer surfaces of the third to fifth ribs (frequently second to fourth)	Coracoid process of the scapula	Depresses the shoulder

Table 5.4 Common muscles – innervation, location and needle placement (*cont'd*)

Muscle	Nerve	Division	L2	L3	L4	L5	S1	S2	S3
Iliopsoas (see Fig. A2.45)	Femoral Nerve	posterior	L2	L3					
Sartorius (see Figs A2.46 & A2.47)	Femoral Nerve	posterior	L2	L3					
Rectus Femoris (see Figs A2.46 & A2.48)	Femoral Nerve	posterior	L2	L3	L4				
Vastus Lateralis (see Figs A2.46 & A2.49)	Femoral Nerve	posterior	L2	L3	L4				
Vastus Intermedius (see Figs A2.46 & A2.50)	Femoral Nerve	posterior	L2	L3	L4				
Vastus Medialis (see Figs A2.46 & A2.51)	Femoral Nerve	posterior	L2	L3	L4				
Pectineus (see Fig. A2.52)	Femoral Nerve	posterior	L2	L3					
Adductor Brevis (see Fig. A2.53)	Obturator Nerve	anterior	L2	L3	L4				
Adductor Longus (see Fig. A2.54)	Obturator Nerve	anterior	L2	L3	L4				
Gracilis (see Fig. A2.55)	Obturator Nerve	anterior	L2	L3	L4				

Needle Insertion	Origin	Insertion	Action
3–4 cm lateral to the femoral artery pulse just below the inguinal ligament	Iliac fossa; ala of sacrum, and lumbar spine	Lesser trochanter on the shaft of the femur, anteromedially	Flexes and internally rotates thigh
5–7.5 cm distal to the anterior superior iliac spine along a line to the medial epicondyle of the tibia	Anterior-superior iliac spine	Upper medial side of tibia	Flexes and externally rotates thigh; flexes and rotates leg medially
The anterior thigh midway between the anterior superior iliac spine and the patella	Anterior-inferior iliac spine; posterior-superior rim of acetabulum	Base of patella; tibial tuberosity	Flexes thigh; extends leg
The anterolateral thigh 7.5–10 cm above the patella	Intertrochanteric line; greater trochanter; linea aspera; gluteal tuberosity; lateral inter-muscular septum	Lateral side of patella; tibial tuberosity	Extends leg
The anterior thigh midway between the anterior superior iliac spine and the patella and under the rectus femoris	Upper shaft of femur; lower lateral intermuscular septum	Upper border of patella; tibial tuberosity	Extends leg
The anteromedial thigh 5–7.5 cm above the patella	Intertrochanteric line; linea aspera; medial intermuscular septum	Medial side of patella; tibial tuberosity	Extends leg
2.5 cm medial to the femoral artery pulse just below the inguinal ligament	Superior ramus of the pubis	Along a line from the lesser trochanter to the linea aspera of the femur	Adducts and flexes thigh
In the proximal 1/6 of the thigh, one-quarter the distance from the medial border to the anterior border of the thigh	Body and inferior pubic ramus	Pectineal line; upper part of linea aspera	Adducts, flexes, and externally rotates thigh
In the proximal 1/5 of the thigh, one-quarter the distance from the medial border to the anterior border of the thigh	Body of pubis below its crest	Middle third of linea aspera	Adducts, flexes, and externally rotates thigh
The junction of the upper and middle thirds of the thigh, along the medial aspect of the thigh	Body and inferior pubic of ramus	Medial surface of upper quarter of tibia	Adducts and flexes thigh; flexes and internally rotates thigh

Table 5.4 Common muscles – innervation, location and needle placement (*cont'd*)

Muscle	Nerve	Division	L2	L3	L4	L5	S1	S2	S3
Adductor Magnus (see Fig. A2.56)	Obturator and Sciatic Nerve	anterior	L2	L3	L4				
Gluteus Medius (see Fig. A2.57)	Superior Gluteal Nerve	posterior			L4	L5	S1		
Gluteus Minimus (see Fig. A2.58)	Superior Gluteal Nerve	posterior			L4	L5	S1		
Tensor Fasciae Latae (see Fig. A2.59)	Superior Gluteal Nerve	posterior			L4	L5	S1		
Gluteus Maximus (see Fig. A2.60)	Inferior Gluteal Nerve	posterior				L5	S1	S2	
Semitendinosus (see Fig. A2.61)	Sciatic Nerve	anterior (tibial portion)				L5	S1	S2	
Semi-membranosus (see Fig. A2.62)	Sciatic Nerve	anterior (tibial portion)				L5	S1	S2	
Biceps Femoris (see Fig. A2.63)	Tibial Nerve (long head) and Common Peroneal Nerve (short head) divisions of Sciatic Nerve	anterior and posterior				L5	S1	S2	
Extensor Digitorum Longus (see Fig. A2.64)	Deep Peroneal Nerve	posterior				L5	S1		
Tibialis Anterior (see Fig. A2.65)	Deep Peroneal Nerve	posterior			L4	L5			

Needle Insertion	Origin	Insertion	Action
Upper one-third of thigh, immediately posterior to the medial border of the thigh	Ischiopubic ramus; ischial tuberosity	Linea aspera; medial supracondylar line; adductor tubercle	Adducts, flexes, and extends thigh
2.5 cm distal to the mid-point of the iliac crest	Superolateral surface of ilium	Greater trochanter	Abducts and aids internal rotation of thigh
Midway between the iliac crest and the greater trochanter of the femur	Ilium between anterior and inferior gluteal lines	Greater trochanter	Abducts and aids internal rotation of thigh
Midway between the anterior superior iliac spine and the greater trochanter of the femur	Iliac crest; anterior - superior iliac spine	Iliotibial tract	Flexes, abducts, and internally rotates thigh
Midpoint of the line connecting the posterior inferior iliac spine and greater trochanter	Posterosuperior ilium and sacrum	Gluteal tuberosity of femur and iliotibial tract	Extends, abducts, and externally rotates thigh
One-third to midway along a line connecting the semitendinosus tendon (easily palpable as it forms the proximal medial margin of the popliteal fossa) with the ischial tuberosity.	Ischial tuberosity	Medial surface of upper part of tibia	Extends thigh; flexes and rotates leg medially
Mid-thigh, at or just medial to the midline and immediately subcutaneous	Ischial tuberosity	Medial condyle of tibia	Extends thigh; flexes and rotates leg medially
Long head: one-third to midway along a line connecting the fibular head with the ischial tuberosity. Short head: Palpate the tendon of the long head of the biceps femoris in the popliteal fossa. Insert the needle just medial to the tendon	Long head from ischial tuberosity; short head from linea aspera and upper supracondylar line	Head of fibula	Extends thigh; flexes and rotates leg medially
5–7.5 cm distal to the tibial tuberosity and 4–5 cm lateral to the shaft of the tibia	Lateral condyle of tibia, interosseous membrane, and fibula	Bases of middle and distal phalanges	Extends toes; dorsiflexes foot
Just lateral to the proximal half of the shaft of the tibia	Proximal half of anterior tibial interosseous membrane and Lateral tibial condyle	Medial (first) cuneiform bone and base of first metatarsal	Dorsiflexes and inverts ankle

Table 5.4 Common muscles – innervation, location and needle placement (*cont'd*)

Muscle	Nerve	Division	L2	L3	L4	L5	S1	S2	S3
Extensor Hallucis Longus (see Fig. A2.66)	Deep Peroneal Nerve	posterior				L5	S1		
Peroneus Tertius (see Fig. A2.67)	Deep Peroneal Nerve	posterior				L5	S1		
Extensor Digitorum Brevis (see Fig. A2.68)	Deep Peroneal Nerve	posterior				L5	S1		
Peroneus Longus (see Fig. A2.69)	Superficial Peroneal Nerve	posterior (peroneal division of Sciatic Nerve)				L5	S1		
Peroneus Brevis (see Fig. A2.70)	Superficial Peroneal Nerve	posterior (peroneal) division of Sciatic Nerve				L5	S1		
Lateral Gastrocnemius (see Fig. A2.71)	Tibial Nerve	anterior				L5	S1		
Medial Gastrocnemius (see Fig. A2.71)	Tibial Nerve	anterior					S1	S2	
Popliteus (see Fig. A2.72)	Tibial Nerve	anterior			L4	L5	S1		
Soleus (see Fig. A2.73)	Tibial Nerve	anterior					S1	S2	
Tibialis Posterior (see Fig. A2.74)	Tibial Nerve	anterior			L4	L5	S1		

Needle Insertion	Origin	Insertion	Action
Approximately 8 cm proximal to the bimalleolar line of the ankle just lateral to the shaft of the tibia	Middle half of anterior surface of fibula; interosseous membrane	Base of distal phalanx of big toe	Extends big toe; dorsiflexes and inverts foot
Approximately 7 cm proximal to the bimalleolar line of the ankle and 2–3 cm lateral to the shaft of the tibia	Distal one-third of fibula; interosseous membrane	Base of fifth metatarsal	Dorsiflexes and everts foot
The superficial muscle tissue located on the proximal lateral aspect of the dorsum of the foot	Calcaneus, lateral talocalcaneal ligament and apex of interior extensor retinaculum	Extensor hood of second to fourth toes	Assists in extension of all toes except little toe
5–7.5 cm below the fibular head along the lateral aspect of the fibula	Lateral tibial condyle; head and upper lateral side of fibula	Medial cuneiform bone and base of first metatarsal	Everts and plantar flexes foot
9–10 cm above the lateral malleolus just posterior to the lateral aspect of the fibula	Lower lateral side of fibula; intermuscular septa	Base of fifth metatarsal foot	Everts and plantar flexes
The midpoint of the lateral mass of the calf	Posterior surface of lateral femoral condyle	Calcaneus	Plantar flexes foot
Midpoint of the medial mass of the calf	Posterior surface of medial femoral condyles	Calcaneus	Plantar flexes foot
The floor of the popliteal fossa in the proximal leg midway between the insertions of the outer and inner hamstring tendons	Lateral femoral condyle	Medially on proximal posterior tibia	Medially rotates and flexes knee
Just distal to the belly of the medial gastrocnemius, medial to the Achilles tendon	Proximal tibia, interosseous membrane, and fibula	Calcaneus	Plantar flexes ankle
1 cm medial to the margin of the tibia at the junction of the upper two-thirds with the lower third of the shaft; direct the needle obliquely through the soleus and flexor digitorum muscles	Posterior shafts of tibia, fibula, and interosseous membrane	Navicular and medial cuneiform bones	Plantar flexes and inverts foot

Table 5.4 Common muscles – innervation, location and needle placement (*cont'd*)

Muscle	Nerve	Division	L2	L3	L4	L5	S1	S2	S3
Flexor Hallucis Longus (see Fig. A2.75)	Tibial Nerve	Anterior				L5	S1	S2	
Abductor Digiti Minimi (see Fig. A2.76)	Lateral Plantar	Anterior					S1	S2	S3
Flexor digiti Minimi (see Fig. A2.77)	Lateral Plantar of Tibial Nerve	Anterior					S1	S2	
Dorsal Interossei (see Fig. A2.78)	Lateral Plantar Nerve (Tibial Nerve)	Anterior						S2	S3
Plantar Interossei (see Fig. A2.79)	Lateral Plantar Nerve (Tibial Nerve)	Anterior						S2	S3
Adductor Hallucis (see Fig. A2.80)	Lateral Plantar Nerve (Tibial Nerve)	Anterior					S1	S2	S3
Abductor Hallucis (see Fig. A2.81)	Medial Plantar Nerve (Tibial Nerve)	Anterior					S1	S2	
Flexor Digitorum Brevis (see Fig. A2.82)	Medial Plantar Nerve (Tibial Nerve)	Anterior					S1	S2	
Flexor Hallucis Brevis (see Fig. A2.83)	Medial Plantar Nerve (Tibial Nerve)	Anterior					S1	S2	

Needle Insertion	Origin	Insertion	Action
The posterolateral aspect of the leg, at the junction of the upper two-thirds with the lower third	Lower two-thirds of fibula; interosseous membrane; intermuscular septa	Base of distal phalanx of big toe	Flexes distal phalanx of big toe
Along the lateral border of the foot midway between the fifth metatarsal head and the calcaneus	Calcaneus	Lateral side of first phalanx of fifth toe	Abducts fifth toe
On plantar aspect of foot, midway between the cuboid and navicular bones	Base of fifth metatarsal	Base of first phalanx of fifth toe	Flexes proximal phalanx of fifth toe
On dorsum of foot, between the metatarsals	Adjacent shafts of metatarsals	Proximal phalanges of second toes (medial and lateral sides), and third and fourth toes (lateral sides)	Abduct toes; flex proximal, and extend distal phalanges
On plantar aspect of foot, between the metatarsals	Medial sides of metatarsals 3–5	Medial sides of base of proximal phalanges 3–5	Adduct toes; flex proximal, and extend distal phalanges
4–5 cm proximal to the second metatarsal head on the plantar surface of the foot to a depth of 2 cm or more (the muscle lies deep); this will access the thick, fleshy oblique head	Oblique head: Bases of metatarsals 2–4 Transverse head: Capsule of lateral four metatarso-phalangeal joints	Proximal phalanx of big toe	Adducts big toe
The muscle belly directly beneath the navicular bone	Medial tubercle of calcaneus	Base of proximal phalanx of big toe	Abducts big toe
Midway between the third metatarsal head and the calcaneus on the plantar surface of the foot	Medial tubercle of calcaneus	Middle phalanges of lateral four toes	Flexes middle phalanx of second through fifth toes
The plantar surface of the foot 2.5 cm proximal to the first metatarsal head	Cuboid; third cuneiform	Proximal phalanx of big toe	Flexes big toe

Table 5.4 Common muscles – innervation, location and needle placement (*cont'd*)

Muscle	Spinal Nerve	Needle Insertion	Action
Paraspinal Muscles			
Cervical paraspinal muscles (including multifidus, supraspinalis, interspinales, rectus capitis and obliquus capitis (see Fig. A2.84)	Posterior primary rami of cervical spinal nerves corresponding to the respective level (intermediate muscles may be innervated by multiple levels)	2 cm lateral to the spinous process of the corresponding level. Note that the C7 level is the most prominent spinous process	Extension of the head
Thoracic paraspinal muscles (see Fig. A2.85)	Posterior primary rami of thoracic spinal nerves corresponding to the respective level (intermediate muscle may be innervated by multiple levels)	2 cm lateral to the spinous process of the corresponding level	Extension of the back
Lumbosacral paraspinal muscles (see Fig. A2.86)	Posterior primary rami of lumbar and sacral spinal nerves corresponding to the respective level (intermediate muscles may be innervated by multiple levels)	2 cm lateral to the spinous process of the corresponding level. Note that the L3–L4 intervertebral level is about the level of the posterior, superior iliac crest	Extension of the hip

Reference:
Chung, K.W, Ph.D., Gross Anatomy, 2nd edn Oxford University Press. Pages 1–107.
Leis, A.A,. Atlas of Electromyography, Oxford, New York, Lippicott Williams of Wilkens Pages 1–195.

6

Injury to Peripheral Nerves

Lyn Weiss

Injury to peripheral nerves can be broken down into those affecting the *myelin* and those affecting the *axons*. It is important to remember however, that rarely is the myelin involved without at least some involvement of the axon (and vice versa). It is the electromyographer who diagnoses what type of injury exists, how severe the injury is, and where the injury is located.

The *Seddon Classification of Nerve Injuries* divides nerve injuries into three categories – neurapraxia, axonotmesis and neurotmesis. *Neurapraxia* is defined as conduction block – only the *myelin* is affected. *Axonotmesis* refers to an injury only affecting the nerve's *axons*. The stroma (supporting connective tissues) is intact. *Neurotmesis* refers to a *complete* injury involving the myelin, axon and all the supporting structures.

Demyelinating Injuries

Demyelinating injuries can slow electrical conduction over the entire length of the nerve (uniform demyelination), slow segments of the nerve (segmental demyelination), slow focal areas of the nerve (focal demyelination), or produce conduction block (when focal demyelination is so severe that nerve action potential propagation across that segment does not occur). These changes are described below.

1. *Uniform demyelination* – the entire length of the nerve displays a slower conduction velocity. This is typically seen in hereditary disorders such as Charcot–Marie–Tooth Disease.

2. *Segmental demyelination* – uneven degree of demyelination of different nerve fibers throughout the course of the nerve. This can produce variable slowing of different nerve fibers, which presents as temporal dispersion (Fig. 6.1). For example, in the same nerve some fibers may be conducting at 50 meters/sec, some at 40 meters/sec and some at 30 meters/sec. The sum will be a waveform that has lower amplitude but is more dispersed (wider). Remember that the sum of all the nerve fibers contributes to the shape of the CMAP.

3. *Focal nerve slowing* – localized area of demyelination causing nerve slowing, which presents as a decrease in conduction velocity across the lesion (Fig. 6.2). For example, if someone applies a tourniquet over one part of an arm, the myelin will be compromised only in that one area. The nerve would conduct normally both above and below that area. Conduction velocity would be slowed across the area of demyelination. This occurs frequently in the ulnar nerve about the elbow.

4. *Conduction block* – an area of focal demyelination that is so severe that the action potential cannot propagate through the area of demyelination. This presents as *decreased amplitude* with proximal stimulation since the affected nerve fibers cannot contribute to

Figure 6.1
Segmental
demyelination.

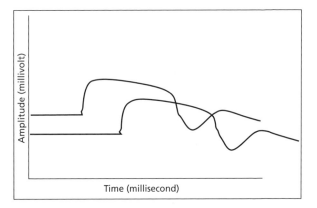

Figure 6.2 Focal
nerve slowing.

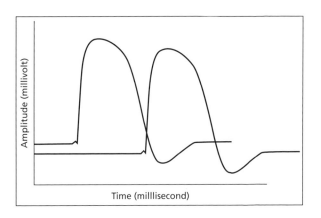

the amplitude. The distal CMAP amplitude is maintained because the nerve fiber distal to the block is intact (Fig. 6.3). For example, if there is a tourniquet applied to the upper arm and the focal demyelination is so severe that the action potential can no longer propagate, the CMAP obtained when stimulating proximal to this point will not include those affected nerve fibers and will therefore have a lower amplitude. However, when the nerve is stimulated distal to this area of compromise, the CMAP will be normal. This is because the axon itself has not been significantly compromised. Clinically, conduction blocks present as weakness. Conduction velocity slowing alone, without conduction block, does not produce clinical weakness.

Because the axon is essentially intact in a purely demyelinating injury, EMG testing will be *normal*, unless conduction block is present. In conduction block, decreased recruitment may be noted.

 ## Axonal Injuries

Injury to the axon will lead to Wallerian degeneration distal to the site of the lesion. In muscles distal to that lesion, you will see a decrease in CMAP amplitude with stimulation, *both* distal and proximal, to the lesion (Fig. 6.4; Fig. 6.5 shows a normal reading for comparison). On needle examination, abnormal spontaneous potentials (fibrillations

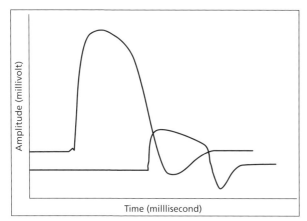

Figure 6.3
Conduction block.

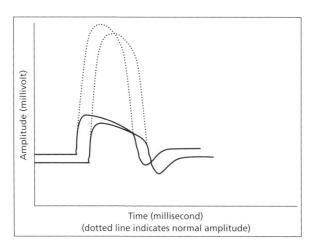

Figure 6.4 Axonal neuropathy.

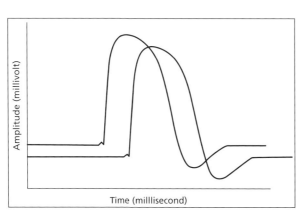

Figure 6.5
Normal.

and positive sharp waves) will be noted. The motor units may be polyphasic with high amplitude and long duration, depending on the chronicity of the injury. Recruitment of motor units will be decreased and firing frequency of single motor units will be increased (normal firing frequency for a MUAP is about 10 Hz or 10 cycles per second).

NCS/EMG Findings

(See Table 6.1)

Nerve Conduction Studies

Demyelinating Injuries

Uniform Demyelinating

In uniform demyelinating lesions nerve conduction studies will be slowed throughout the nerve since the entire nerve is affected. Distal latencies will be prolonged; again because of the uniform slowing (distal latencies representing the most distal conduction velocity). Amplitudes should not be significantly affected, since the axons are intact and the slowing is consistent through all fibers of the nerve.

Segmental Demyelination

Since there is variable slowing of different nerve fibers within the nerve, conduction velocity will be slowed and distal latencies will be prolonged in segmentally demyelinating injuries. CMAP amplitudes will be decreased because of temporal dispersion, not because of axonal damage. Therefore, the CMAP will be longer in duration and the area under the CMAP will be normal.

Focal Demyelination

In focal demyelination, only one segment of the nerve is affected. Therefore, conduction velocity will be normal *unless* stimulation is across the area of focal demyelination. In this segment, you will see slowing of conduction velocity. Slowing is usually evident if there is a more than 10 meter/second drop in conduction velocity across the segment, compared to distally. Latencies and amplitudes should be normal.

Conduction Block

As stated above, conduction block is a *focal* demyelination that is so severe that the action potential cannot propagate past that point. Therefore, distal latencies and conduction velocities remain normal. Distal amplitudes will be normal. However, when the nerve is stimulated *across* the area of conduction block, a drop in amplitude is noted. To be considered significant, this drop in proximal amplitude should be more than 20% of the distal amplitude. For example if the distal amplitude is 10 microvolts and the proximal amplitude is 7 microvolts, conduction block should be considered.

Axonal Injuries

Nerve conduction studies in axonal injuries will show decreased amplitude with *both* proximal and distal stimulation. If the contralateral extremity is not affected, you can compare side-to-side amplitudes to estimate the amount of axonal loss. Usually, a 50% side-to-side difference is considered significant. Latencies and conduction velocities should not be significantly affected. Sometimes, since the fastest fibers may be affected, a less than 20% increase in latency or decrease in conduction velocity may be noted. If

Table 6.1 NCS/EMG findings in peripheral nerve injuries

Condition	CMAP amplitude with distal stimulation	CMAP amplitude with proximal stimulation (stimulating across the lesion)	Conduction velocity	Distal latency	Fibs/PSW	Recruitment
Uniform demyelinating	Normal	Normal	Decreased	Increased	–	Normal
Segmental demyelinating	Normal or decreased secondary to dispersion	Decreased secondary to dispersion	Decreased	May be increased (if fastest fibers are affected)	–	Normal
Focal demyelinating without conduction block*	Normal	Normal	Slowed across area of focal demyelination	Normal	–	Normal
Focal demyelination causing conduction block*	Normal	(Decreased by more than 20%)	Normal or focal slowing	Normal	–	Decreased
Axonotmesis	Decreased	Decreased	Normal to 20% decrease	Normal to 20% increase	+	Decreased
Neurotmesis	Unobtainable	Unobtainable	Unobtainable	Unobtainable	++	Unobtainable

*For the purposes of this table, assume a proximal area of focal demyelination or conduction block.

neurotmesis is present, the CMAP or SNAP amplitude will be unobtainable both proximal and distal to the lesion.

EMG Findings

Abnormal spontaneous potentials (fibrillations and positive sharp waves) are usually only found if there has been axonal injury. Therefore, no abnormal spontaneous activity should be noted in any of the *demyelinating lesions*. MUAP morphology and recruitment should be normal. The only exception would be in conduction block, where decreased recruitment would be seen.

With Wallerian degeneration, the degeneration occurs *distal* to the site of the lesion. Therefore, all distal muscles innervated by the injured nerve should show spontaneous activity *if* the test is performed before reinnervation occurs (see below). Polyphasicity, prolonged duration and increased amplitude of the MUAP may be noted, again depending upon the timing of the test. Recruitment will be decreased. In a neurotmetic lesion, there will be profound denervation and no motor units will be recruited.

Timing of Electrodiagnostic Testing – When to Schedule an EMG/NCS

In order to get the most information with the least amount of discomfort to the patient, it is important to time the test appropriately. Keep in mind the following timetable regarding how nerves respond electrophysiologically to injury:

1. Abnormal spontaneous activity includes fibrillation potentials (fibs) and positive sharp waves (PSWs). Such findings may take days to weeks before being detectable on EMG testing. The more distal the muscle, the longer the axon length, and the longer it takes for membrane instability to occur. Proximal muscles may show changes within one week, but collateral sprouting will also provide reinnervation to these muscles first. More distal muscles may require *three weeks* before fibs or PSWs are seen. Therefore, if the test is done too early (e.g., in the first few weeks after injury) it may be falsely negative. If a test is performed long after the injury, reinnervation may have already occurred. In this case, there may not be fibs and PSWs present. Motor units may show evidence of reinnervation – long duration, polyphasic and increased amplitude.

2. Sensory nerve action potentials (SNAPs) and compound muscle action potentials (CMAPs) amplitudes begin to decrease within several days after nerve injury. It may take over one week before SNAPs and CMAPs are unobtainable. Therefore, if NCS are done in the first few days after injury, they may appear normal when in fact, if they were done at least *11 days* following the injury, they would reveal reduced amplitudes consistent with the suspected injury.

3. Axons regrow at a rate of about 1 mm/day (about an inch per month). Therefore, if you are doing a study or serial studies where you want to determine the prognosis, it is important to keep in mind how long the anticipated recovery period would be based on axonal regeneration.

7

How to Plan Out the Examination

Lyn Weiss, Carlo Esteves, Limeng Wang

To perform electrodiagnostic testing accurately and efficiently, a well-planned approach is necessary. Such measures will decrease potential discomfort and increase the yield of information. The clinician should start by taking a thorough history, performing a physical examination and, if available, reviewing laboratory and radiological studies. Electrodiagnostic testing serves as an adjunct to the history and physical examination in the evaluation of neuromuscular disease/pathology. Although the nature of neurologic dysfunction in a specific disease process may be suggested by symptoms or signs obtained during physical examination, only electrodiagnostic studies can provide an objective physiologic measure of neurologic function.

Once the history and physical are performed, you should develop a differential diagnosis that will help guide which nerves and muscles are tested. There are several questions that can help you narrow your selections (Fig. 7.1).

- Are the symptoms compatible with a central disorder (hyperreflexia, increased tone, central distribution) or a peripheral disorder (hyporeflexia, decreased tone, peripheral distribution)? If the history and physical are compatible with a central disorder, other testing may be more appropriate (i.e., MRI of the brain or spinal cord). If a peripheral distribution is suggested, proceed with EMG/NCS testing.
- Does the history and physical suggest a disorder of nerves (neuropathic) or muscles (myopathic)? A neuropathic disorder may present with sensory findings and/or weakness in a peripheral nerve distribution. A myopathic disorder should be considered if there is predominantly proximal weakness and no sensory symptoms (see Chapter 17).
- If a neuropathic disorder is more likely, try to determine if the motor and sensory loss reflects a peripheral neuropathy (predominantly distal affecting more than one extremity) or a peripheral nerve distribution.
- If a peripheral nerve lesion is probable, use Table 7.1 to try to localize the lesion. Table 7.1 will help you identify the patient's symptoms, depending on whether the problem is at the root, trunk, cord division or peripheral nerve level. It will also help you determine which nerves and muscles should be tested.
- If a peripheral neuropathy is suspected, electrodiagnostic testing will help determine the type of neuropathy (motor and/or sensory; axonal and/or demyelinating).

General Points to Remember

- If you get an abnormal result, it is important to continue testing until you get a normal result. For example, if you suspect carpal tunnel syndrome and the needle

Figure 7.1
Algorithm for
planning the
electrodiagnostic
examination.

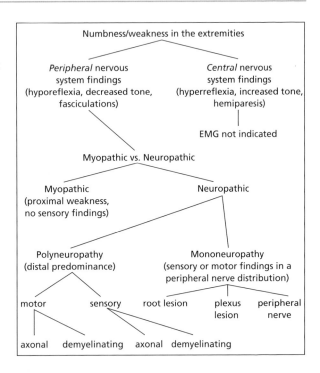

testing of the abductor pollicis brevis (APB) is abnormal (fibrillations or positive sharp waves are present), other muscles should be tested. A more proximal median neuropathy may be present, or a generalized disorder may be present.

- To assess for peripheral neuropathy, motor and sensory nerves in two or three extremities must be tested.
- When performing needle testing to rule out local nerve injury or entrapment, start with the most distally innervated muscles and proceed proximally.
- If the patient is reluctant to proceed with the electrodiagnostic test, go directly to that portion of the test that is most likely to yield pertinent information. For example, some electromyographers have a prescribed list and schedule of nerves to test. While this may suffice for 90% of patients, flexibility is necessary if you know the patient can only tolerate limited testing.

Table 7.1 shows commonly tested nerves in the upper and lower extremities, the root levels, the muscles they innervate, and some of the physical findings that can be expected if the nerve is compromised. This table can be used to help plan out the electrodiagnostic test. Table 7.2 describes common muscles tested on needle study, along with nerve and root levels. This will assist with planning out the examination. For example, if a C6 nerve root is suspected, try to examine several muscles that include C6. If a radial nerve injury is suspected, these tables will help decide which muscles to test based on their innervation.

Table 7.1 Upper extremities

Roots	Nerves	Muscles	Root lesion Signs and symptoms
C5	Dorsal scapular	Rhomboid major	Weakness or absent scapula adduction.
	Dorsal scapular	Rhomboid minor	Weakness in shoulder range of motion.
	Dorsal scapular	Levator scapulae	Weakness in arm abduction, adduction, flexion and medial/lateral rotation.
	Suprascapular	Supraspinatus	Weakness in flexion of forearm at elbow and supination of forearm.
	Suprascapular	Infraspinatus	Diminished sensation over the lateral arm
	Subscapular	Subscapularis	
	Subscapular	Teres major	
	Axillary	Deltoid	
	Axillary	Teres minor	
	Musculocutaneous	Coracobrachialis	
	Musculocutaneous	Biceps	
	Musculocutaneous	Brachialis	
	Long thoracic	Serratus anterior	
	Radial	Brachioradialis	
	Radial	Supinator	
	Pectoral	Pectoralis major	
	Pectoral	Pectoralis minor	
C6	Suprascapular	Supraspinatus	Weakness in arm abduction, adduction, flexion and medial/lateral rotation.
	Suprascapular	Infraspinatus	Weakness in extension/flexion of forearm at elbow and pronation of forearm.
	Subscapular	Subscapularis	Weakness in extension (dorsiflexion) wrist and radial abduction of hand at wrist.
	Subscapular	Teres major	Diminished sensation over the lateral forearm, thumb, index, and one-half of middle finger (radial side)
	Axillary	Deltoid	
	Axillary	Teres minor	
	Musculocutaneous	Biceps	
	Musculocutaneous	Brachialis	
	Musculocutaneous	Coracobrachialis	
	Thoracodorsal	Latissimus dorsi	
	Long thoracic	Serratus anterior	

Table 7.1 Upper extremities (cont'd)

Roots	Nerves	Muscles	Root lesion Signs and symptoms
	Radial	Triceps	
	Radial	Anconeus	
	Radial	Brachioradialis	
	Radial	Extensor carpi radialis	
	Radial	Supinator	
	Median	Pronator teres	
	Median	Flexor carpi radialis	
	Pectoral	Pectoralis major	
	Pectoral	Pectoralis minor	
C7	Subscapular	Teres major	Weak or absent extension of forearm at elbow and pronation of forearm.
	Musculocutaneous	Coracobrachialis	Unable to flex (palmar flexion) hand at wrist and extend fingers at MCP.
	Thoracodorsal	Latissimus dorsi	Inability to dorsiflex the wrist and ulnar deviation.
	Long thoracic	Serratus anterior	Weakness in extension (dorsiflexion) wrist and radial abduction of hand at wrist.
	Radial	Triceps	Weakness in extension of proximal and distal phalanx of thumb.
	Radial	Anconeus	Diminished sensation over middle finger
	Radial	Extensor carpi radialis	
	Radial	Extensor carpi ulnaris	
	Radial	Extensor digitorum	
	Radial	Extensor digiti minimi	
	Radial	Abductor pollicis longus	
	Radial	Extensor pollicis longus	
	Radial	Extensor pollicis brevis	
	Radial	Extensor indicis	
	Median	Pronator teres	
	Median	Flexor carpi radialis	
	Median	Palmaris longus	
	Median	Flexor digitorum superficialis	
	Median and ulnar	Flexor digitorum profundus	

Table 7.1 Upper extremities (cont'd)

Roots	Nerves	Muscles	Root lesion Signs and symptoms
	Median	Flexor pollicis longus	
	Median	Pronator quadratus	
	Pectoral	Pectoralis major	
	Pectoral	Pectoralis minor	
C8	Radial	Extensor carpi ulnaris	Weakness in flexion of distal phalanges of fingers.
	Radial	Extensor digitorum	Inability to adduct index, ring and little fingers towards middle finger.
	Radial	Extensor digiti minimi	Difficulty of abduction of index, middle and ring finger from middle line of middle
	Radial	Abductor pollicis longus	finger both radial and ulnar abduction.
	Radial	Extensor pollicis longus	Weakness in flexion and ulnar deviation of hand at wrist.
	Radial	Extensor pollicis brevis	Weakness in abduction, flexion and opposition of little finger towards thumb.
	Radial	Extensor indicis	Unable to adduct the thumb in both ulnar and palmar directions.
	Median	Palmaris longus	Diminished sensation over the distal half of the forearm's ulnar side, the 5th and
	Median	Flexor digitorum superficialis	half of the 4th finger on the ulnar side
	Median and ulnar	Flexor digitorum profundus	
	Median	Flexor pollicis longus	
	Median	Pronator quadratus	
	Median	Abductor pollicis brevis	
	Median	Opponens pollicis	
	Median	Flexor pollicis brevis	
	Ulnar	Flexor carpi ulnaris	
	Ulnar	Palmaris brevis	
	Ulnar	Abductor digiti minimi	
	Ulnar	Opponens digiti minimi	
	Ulnar	Flexor digiti minimi	
	Ulnar	Palmar interosseous	
	Ulnar	Dorsal interosseous	

Table 7.1 Upper extremities (cont'd)

Roots	Nerves	Muscles	Root lesion Signs and symptoms
	Ulnar	Adductor pollicis	
	Median and ulnar	Lumbricals (4)	
	Pectoral	Pectoralis major	
	Pectoral	Pectoralis minor	
T1	Median	Palmaris longus	Weakness in finger abduction. Difficulty of abduction of index, middle and ring finger from middle line of middle finger both radial and ulnar abduction.
	Median	Flexor digitorum superficialis	Inability to adduct index, ring and little fingers towards middle finger.
	Median and ulnar	Flexor digitorum profundus	Weakness in little finger abduction, flexion and opposition of little finger towards thumb.
	Median	Flexor pollicis longus	Weakness in adduction of the thumb in both ulnar and palmar directions and abduction of thumb.
	Median	Pronator quadratus	Diminished sensation over the medial side of the upper half of the forearm and the lower half of the arm.
	Median	Abductor pollicis brevis	
	Median	Opponens pollicis	
	Median	Flexor pollicis brevis	
	Ulnar	Flexor carpi ulnaris	
	Ulnar	Palmaris brevis	
	Ulnar	Abductor digiti minimi	
	Ulnar	Opponens digiti minimi	
	Ulnar	Flexor digiti minimi	
	Ulnar	Palmar interosseous	
	Ulnar	Dorsal interosseous	
	Ulnar	Adductor pollicis	
	Median and ulnar	Lumbricals (4)	
	Pectoral	Pectoralis major	
	Pectoral	Pectoralis minor	

Table 7.1 Upper extremities (cont'd).

Trunks	Nerves	Muscles	Trunk lesion Signs and symptoms
Upper trunk C5, C6	Dorsal scapula	Rhomboid major	Weakness of shoulder and upper arm abduction, flexion, and external rotation.
	Dorsal scapula	Rhomboid minor	Weakness in elbow flexion and radial wrist extension.
	Dorsal scapula	Levator scapulae	Sensory loss at the C5 and C6 dermatomes – the lateral arm, forearm, and first two digits
	Suprascapular	Supraspinatus	
	Suprascapular	Infraspinatus	
	Suprascapular	Subscapularis	
	Suprascapular	Teres major	
	Axillary	Deltoid	
	Axillary	Teres minor	
	Musculocutaneous	Coracobrachialis	
	Musculocutaneous	Biceps	
	Musculocutaneous	Brachialis	
	Thoracodorsal	Latissimus dorsi	
	Radial	Triceps	
	Radial	Anconeus	
	Radial	Brachioradialis	
	Radial	Extensor carpi radialis	
	Radial	Supinator	
	Median	Pronator teres	
	Median	Flexor carpi radialis	
	Pectoral	Pectoralis major	
	Pectoral	Pectoralis minor	
Middle trunk C7	Musculocutaneous	Coracobrachialis	Weak or absent extension of forearm at elbow.
	Thoracodorsal	Latissimus dorsi	Weak/absent extension (dorsiflexion) and radial abduction of hand at wrist. Unable to flex (palmar flexion) hand at wrist and extend fingers at MCP.
	Radial	Triceps	Inability to dorsiflex the wrist and ulnar deviation.
	Radial	Anconeus	Weak or absent extension of proximal and distal phalanx of thumb.
	Radial	Extensor carpi radialis	Diminished sensation over middle finger and sometimes the index finger
	Radial	Extensor carpi ulnaris	

Table 7.1 Upper extremities (cont'd)

Trunks	Nerves	Muscles	Trunk lesion Signs and symptoms
	Radial	Extensor digitorum	
	Radial	Extensor digiti minimi	
	Radial	Abductor pollicis longus	
	Radial	Extensor pollicis longus	
	Radial	Extensor pollicis brevis	
	Radial	Extensor indicis	
	Median	Pronator teres	
	Median	Flexor carpi radialis	
	Median	Palmaris longus	
	Median	Flexor digitorum superficialis	
	Median and ulnar	Flexor digitorum profundus	
	Median	Flexor pollicis longus	
	Median	Pronator quadratus	
	Pectoral	Pectoralis major	
	Pectoral	Pectoralis minor	
Lower trunk C8, T1	Thoracodorsal	Latissimus dorsi	Weak or absent abduction, flexion and opposition of little finger towards thumb.
	Radial	Triceps	Inability to adduct index, ring and little fingers towards middle finger.
	Radial	Anconeus	Difficulty of abduction of index, middle and ring finger from middle line of middle finger both radial and ulnar abduction.
	Radial	Extensor carpi ulnaris	Unable to adduct the thumb in both ulnar and palmar directions.
	Radial	Extensor digitorum	Weakness in extension of forearm and flexion of distal phalanges.
	Radial	Extensor digiti minimi	Diminished sensation over distal half of the forearm ulnar side, the 5th and half of the 4th finger on the ulnar side
	Radial	Abductor pollicis longus	
	Radial	Extensor pollicis longus	
	Radial	Extensor pollicis brevis	
	Radial	Extensor indicis	
	Median	Palmaris longus	
	Median	Flexor digitorum superficialis	
	Median and ulnar	Flexor digitorum profundus	

Table 7.1 Upper extremities (cont'd)

Trunks	Nerves	Muscles	Trunk lesion Signs and symptoms
	Median	Flexor pollicis longus	
	Median	Pronator quadratus	
	Ulnar	Abductor digiti minimi	
	Ulnar	Opponens digiti minimi	
	Ulnar	Flexor digiti minimi	
	Ulnar	Palmar interosseous	
	Ulnar	Dorsal interosseous	
	Ulnar	Adductor pollicis	
	Median and ulnar	Lumbricals (4)	
	Pectoral	Pectoralis major	
	Pectoral	Pectoralis minor	

Cords	Nerves	Muscles	Cord lesion Signs and symptoms
Posterior cord C5 to T1	Subscapular	Subscapularis	Weakness in shoulder ROM and arm abduction, adduction, flexion, extension, lateral rotation.
	Subscapular	Teres major	Weak or absent extension of forearm at elbow.
	Axillary	Deltoid	Weak or absent extension (dorsiflexion) and radial abduction of hand at wrist.
	Axillary	Teres minor	Unable to supinate and extend fingers at MCP.
	Thoracodorsal	Latissimus dorsal	Inability to dorsiflex the wrist and ulnar deviation.
	Radial	Triceps	Weak or absent extension of proximal and distal phalanx of thumb.
	Radial	Anconeus	Diminished sensation over the lateral arm – deltoid patch on upper arm, lateral forearm and first 3 digits
	Radial	Brachioradialis	
	Radial	Extensor carpi radialis	
	Radial	Supinator	
	Radial	Extensor carpi ulnaris	
	Radial	Extensor digitorum	
	Radial	Extensor digiti minimi	
	Radial	Abductor pollicis longus	
	Radial	Extensor pollicis longus	

Table 7.1 Upper extremities (cont'd)

Cords	Nerves	Muscles	Cord lesion Signs and symptoms
	Radial	Extensor pollicis brevis	
	Radial	Extensor indicis	
Lateral cord C5 to T1	Musculocutaneous	Coracobrachialis	Unable to pronate and flex the forearm.
	Musculocutaneous	Biceps	Weakness in flexion of forearms and the hand at wrist.
	Musculocutaneous	Brachialis	Weakness in flexion of distal phalanges of fingers.
	Median	Pronator teres	Diminished sensation over the lateral forearm and middle finger
	Median	Flexor carpi radialis	
	Median	Palmaris longus	
	Median	Flexor digitorum superficialis	
	Median and ulnar	Flexor digitorum profundus	
	Median	Flexor pollicis longus	
	Pectoral	Pectoralis major	
	Pectoral	Pectoralis minor	
Medial cord C6 to T1	Median	Palmaris longus	Weakness in flexion of distal phalanges of fingers.
	Median	Flexor digitorum superficialis	Weak/absent abduction, flexion and opposition of little finger towards thumb.
	Median and ulnar	Flexor digitorum profundus	Inability to adduct index, ring and little fingers towards middle finger. Difficulty of abduction of index, middle and ring fingers from middle line of middle finger both radial and ulnar abduction.
	Median	Flexor pollicis longus	Unable to adduct the thumb in both ulnar and palmar directions.
	Median	Pronator quadratus	Decreased sensation over the volar surface of the 1st to 3rd and half of the
	Median	Abductor pollicis brevis	4th fingers
	Median	Opponens pollicis	
	Median	Flexor pollicis brevis	
	Ulnar	Flexor carpi ulnaris	
	Ulnar	Palmaris brevis	

Table 7.1 Upper extremities (cont'd)

Cords	Nerves	Muscles	Cord lesion Signs and symptoms
	Ulnar	Abductor digiti minimi	
	Ulnar	Opponens digiti minimi	
	Ulnar	Flexor digiti minimi	
	Ulnar	Palmar interosseous	
	Ulnar	Dorsal interosseous	
	Ulnar	Adductor pollicis	
	Median and ulnar	Lumbricals (4)	

Divisions	Nerves	Muscles	Division lesion Signs and symptoms
Posterior division C5 to C8	Subscapular	Subscapularis	Weakness in shoulder ROM and arm abduction, adduction, flexion, extension, lateral rotation.
	Subscapular	Teres major	
	Axillary	Deltoid	Weak or absent extension of forearm at elbow.
	Axillary	Teres minor	Weak or absent extension (dorsiflexion) and radial abduction of hand at wrist.
	Thoracodorsal	Latissimus dorsi	Unable to supinate and extend fingers at MCP.
	Radial	Triceps	Inability to dorsiflex the wrist and ulnar deviation.
	Radial	Anconeus	Weak or absent extension of proximal and distal phalanx of thumb.
	Radial	Brachioradialis	Diminished sensation over the lateral arm – deltoid patch on upper arm, lateral forearm and first 3 digits
	Radial	Extensor carpi radialis	
	Radial	Supinator	
	Radial	Extensor carpi ulnaris	
	Radial	Extensor digitorum	
	Radial	Extensor digiti minimi	
	Radial	Abductor pollicis longus	
	Radial	Extensor pollicis longus	
	Radial	Extensor pollicis brevis	
	Radial	Extensor indicis	

Table 7.1 Upper extremities (cont'd)

Divisions	Nerves	Muscles	Division lesion / Signs and symptoms
Anterior division C5 to T1	Musculocutaneous	Coracobrachialis	Weakness or absent supination of forearm and flexion of forearm at elbow.
	Musculocutaneous	Biceps	Numbness/tingling sensation on the volar surface of the 1st to 3rd and half of the 4th fingers.
	Musculocutaneous	Brachialis	Weak/absent palmar abduction of thumb (perpendicular to plane of palm).
	Median	Pronator teres	Weakness in flexion of distal phalanges of fingers.
	Median	Flexor carpi radialis	Weak/absent abduction, flexion and opposition of little finger towards thumb.
	Median	Palmaris longus	Inability to adduct index, ring and little fingers towards middle finger.
	Median	Flexor digitorum superficialis	Difficulty of abduction of index, middle and ring fingers from middle line of middle finger both radial and ulnar directions.
	Median and ulnar	Flexor digitorum profundus	Unable to adduct the thumb in both ulnar and palmar directions.
	Median	Flexor pollicis longus	Diminished sensation over the lateral forearm, 3rd, 4th, and 5th fingers
	Median	Pronator quadratus	
	Median	Abductor pollicis brevis	
	Median	Opponens pollicis	
	Median	Flexor pollicis brevis	
	Ulnar	Flexor carpi ulnaris	
	Ulnar	Palmaris brevis	
	Ulnar	Abductor digiti minimi	
	Ulnar	Opponens digiti minimi	
	Ulnar	Flexor digiti minimi	
	Ulnar	Palmar interosseous	
	Ulnar	Dorsal interosseous	
	Ulnar	Adductor pollicis	
	Median and ulnar	Lumbricals (4)	
	Pectoral	Pectoralis major	
	Pectoral	Pectoralis minor	

Table 7.1 Upper extremities (cont'd)

Peripheral nerves	Roots	Muscles	Peripheral nerve lesion Signs and symptoms
Axillary	C5, C5, C5, C6	Deltoid Teres minor	Weakness in shoulder range of motion and arm abduction, adduction, flexion, extension, lateral rotation. Diminished sensation over the lateral arm – deltoid patch on upper arm
Musculocutaneous	C5, C6, C7 C5, C6 C5, C6	Coracobrachialis Biceps Brachialis	Weakness or absent supination of forearm and flexion of forearm at elbow. Decreased sensory over the lateral forearm
Radial	C6, C7, C8 C6, C7, C8 C5, C6 C6, C7 C5, C6 C7, C8 C7, C8 C7, C8 C7, C8 C7, C8 C7, C8 C7, C8	Triceps Anconeus Brachioradialis Extensor carpi radialis Supinator Extensor carpi ulnaris Extensor digitorum Extensor digiti minimi Abductor pollicis longus Extensor pollicis longus Extensor pollicis brevis Extensor indicis	Weak or absent extension of forearm at elbow. Weak or absent extension (dorsiflexion) and radial abduction of hand at wrist. Unable to supinate and extend fingers at MCP. Inability to dorsiflex the wrist and ulnar deviation. Weak or absent extension of proximal and distal phalanx of thumb. Sensation is diminished over the web space between thumb and index finger
Median	C6, C7 C6, C7 C7, C8, T1 C7, C8, T1 C7, C8, T1 C7, C8, T1 C7, C8, T1 C8, T1	Pronator teres Flexor carpi radialis Palmaris longus Flexor digitorum superficialis Flexor digitorum profundus Flexor pollicis longus Pronator quadratus Abductor pollicis brevis	Unable to pronate the forearm and flex the hand at wrist. Numbness/tingling sensation on the volar surface of the 1st to 3rd and half of the 4th fingers. Weak/absent palmar abduction of thumb (perpendicular to plane of palm). Unable to do the 'OK' sign. Decreased sensation over the distal radial aspect index finger

Table 7.1 Upper extremities (cont'd)

Peripheral nerves	Roots	Muscles	Peripheral nerve lesion Signs and symptoms
	C8, T1	Opponens pollicis	
	C8, T1	Flexor pollicis brevis	
	C8, T1	Lumbricals	
Ulnar nerve	C8, T1	Flexor carpi ulnaris	Weak/absent abduction, flexion and opposition of little finger towards thumb.
	C8, T1	Flexor digitorum profundus	Inability to adduct index, ring and little fingers towards middle finger.
	C8, T1	Palmaris brevis	Difficulty of abduction of index, middle and ring fingers from middle line of middle finger both radial and ulnar abduction.
	C8, T1	Abductor digiti minimi	Unable to adduct the thumb in both ulnar and palmar directions.
	C8, T1	Opponens digiti minimi	Decreased sensory over the 5th and half of the 4th finger on the ulnar side
	C8, T1	Flexor digiti minimi	
	C8, T1	Palmar interosseous	
	C8, T1	Dorsal interosseous	
	C8, T1	Adductor pollicis	
	C8, T1	Flexor pollicis brevis	
	C8, T1	Lumbricals	

Lower extremities

Roots	Nerves	Muscles	Root lesion Signs and symptoms
L2	Femoral	Iliopsoas	Weakness in hip adduction and flexion.
	Femoral	Sartorius	Weak or absent thigh adduction, flexion, medial and lateral rotation.
	Femoral	Rectus femoris	Weakness or inability to extend the leg at the knee.
	Femoral	Vastus lateralis	Diminished sensation over the anterior and medial aspects of the thigh and in the medial aspect of the leg
	Femoral	Vastus intermedius	
	Femoral	Vastus medialis	
	Femoral	Pectineus	
	Obturator	Adductor brevis	
	Obturator	Adductor longus	
	Obturator	Gracilis	
	Obturator	Adductor magnus	

Table 7.1 Lower extremities (cont'd)

Roots	Nerves	Muscles	Lower extremities Root lesion Signs and symptoms
L3	Femoral Femoral Femoral Femoral Femoral Femoral Femoral Obturator Obturator Obturator Obturator	Iliopsoas Sartorius Rectus femoris Vastus lateralis Vastus intermedius Vastus medialis Pectineus Adductor brevis Adductor longus Gracilis Adductor magnus	Weakness in hip adduction and flexion. Weak or absent thigh adduction, flexion, medial and lateral rotation. Weakness or inability to extend the leg at the knee. Diminished sensation over the anterior and medial aspect of the thigh and knee
L4	Femoral Femoral Femoral Femoral Obturator Obturator Obturator Obturator Superior gluteal Superior gluteal Superior gluteal Deep peroneal Tibial	Rectus femoris Vastus lateralis Vastus intermedius Vastus medialis Adductor brevis Adductor longus Gracilis Adductor magnus Gluteus medius Gluteus minimus Tensor fasciae latae Tibialis anterior Popliteus	Weakness in hip adduction and abduction. Weak or absent thigh adduction, abduction, flexion, medial and lateral rotation. Weakness in knee flexion, medial rotation and extension. Loss of dorsiflexion (drop foot). Limited inversion of foot. Diminished sensation over the medial side of the distal leg and medial malleolus area

Table 7.1 Lower extremities (cont'd)

Roots	Nerves	Muscles	Lower extremities Root lesion Signs and symptoms
L5	Superior gluteal	Gluteus medius	Weakness in adduction, abduction, flexion, extension, medial and lateral rotation of thigh.
	Superior gluteal	Gluteus minimus	Weakness in flexion and medial rotation of leg.
	Superior gluteal	Tensor fasciae latae	Loss of dorsiflexion (drop foot).
	Inferior gluteal	Gluteus maximus	Limited inversion/eversion of foot.
	Sciatic	Semitendinosus	Unable to extend all toes.
	Sciatic	Semimembranosus	Weakness or absent plantar flexion of the foot/toes and flexion of the knee.
	Sciatic	Biceps femoris	Diminished sensation over the lateral half of the leg and the dorsum of the foot especially the big toe and the second toe
	Deep peroneal	Extensor digitorum longus	
	Deep peroneal	Tibialis anterior	
	Deep peroneal	Extensor hallucis longus	
	Deep peroneal	Peroneus tertius	
	Deep peroneal	Extensor digitorum brevis	
	Superficial peroneal	Peroneus longus	
	Superficial peroneal	Peroneus brevis	
	Tibial	Popliteus	
	Tibial	Tibialis posterior	
	Tibial	Flexor hallucis longus	
	Tibial	Flexor digitorum longus	
S1	Superior gluteal	Gluteus medius	Weakness in adduction, abduction, flexion, extension, medial and lateral rotation of thigh.
	Superior gluteal	Gluteus minimus	Weakness in flexion and medial rotation of leg.
	Superior gluteal	Tensor fasciae latae	Weakness or absent plantar flexion of the foot/toes and flexion of the knee.
	Inferior gluteal	Gluteus maximus	Loss of dorsiflexion (drop foot).
	Sciatic	Semitendinosus	Limited inversion/eversion of foot.
	Sciatic	Semimembranosus	Unable to extend all toes.
	Sciatic	Biceps femoris	Diminished sensation over the posterior, distal third of the leg, lateral heel, lateral foot and little toe
	Deep peroneal	Extensor digitorum longus	

Table 7.1 Lower extremities (cont'd)

Roots	Nerves	Muscles	Lower extremities Root lesion Signs and symptoms
	Deep peroneal	Extensor hallucis longus	
	Deep peroneal	Peroneus tertius	
	Deep peroneal	Extensor digitorum brevis	
	Superficial peroneal	Peroneus longus	
	Superficial peroneal	Peroneus brevis	
	Tibial	Gastrocnemius	
	Tibial	Popliteus	
	Tibial	Soleus	
	Tibial	Tibialis posterior	
	Tibial	Flexor hallucis longus	
	Tibial	Flexor digitorum longus	
	Tibial	Abductor digiti minimi	
	Tibial	Quadratus plantae	
	Tibial	Flexor digiti minimi	
	Tibial	Lumbricals	
	Tibial	Adductor hallucis	
	Tibial	Abductor hallucis	
	Tibial	Flexor digitorum brevis	
	Tibial	Flexor hallucis brevis	
S2	Inferior gluteal	Gluteus maximus	Weakness or absent plantar flexion of the foot/toes and flexion of the knee. Sensory problem over the posterior area of the leg
	Sciatic	Semitendinosus	
	Sciatic	Semimembranosus	
	Sciatic	Biceps femoris	
	Tibial	Gastrocnemius	
	Tibial	Soleus	
	Tibial	Flexor hallucis longus	
	Tibial	Flexor digitorum longus	
	Tibial	Abductor digiti minimi	

Table 7.1 Lower extremities (cont'd)

Roots	Nerves	Muscles	Lower extremities — Root lesion Signs and symptoms
	Tibial	Quadratus plantae	Weakness or absent plantar flexion of the foot/toes and flexion of the knee.
	Tibial	Flexor digiti minimi	
	Tibial	Lumbricals	
	Tibial	Dorsal interossei	
	Tibial	Plantar interossei	
	Tibial	Adductor hallucis	
	Tibial	Abductor hallucis	
	Tibial	Flexor digitorum brevis	
	Tibial	Flexor hallucis brevis	
S3	Tibial	Abductor digiti minimi	Diminished sensation over the perianal area
	Tibial	Dorsal interossei	
	Tibial	Plantar interossei	
	Tibial	Adductor hallucis	

Plexus	Nerves	Muscles	Plexus lesion Signs and symptoms
Lumbar plexus T12, L1 to L4	Iliohypogastric	Transversus abdominis	Weakness in hip adduction and flexion.
	Iliohypogastric	Internal oblique muscles	Weak or absent thigh adduction, flexion, medial and lateral rotation.
	Iliohypogastric	External oblique muscles	Weakness or inability to extend the leg at the knee.
	Ilioinguinal	Transversus abdominis	Diminished sensation over the upper buttock, scrotum or labium, hypogastric region, anterior, medial and lateral aspect of the thigh, and the medial aspect of the leg
	Ilioinguinal	Internal oblique muscles	
	Genitofemoral	Cremaster	
	L1, L2, L3	Quadratus lumborum	
	L1, L2, L3	Psoas minor	
	L1, L2, L3, L4	Psoas major	
	Femoral	Iliopsoas	
	Femoral	Sartorius	
	Femoral	Rectus femoris	

Table 7.1 Lower extremities (cont'd)

Plexus	Nerves	Muscles	Plexus lesion Signs and symptoms
	Femoral	Vastus lateralis	
	Femoral	Vastus intermedius	
	Femoral	Vastus medialis	
	Femoral	Pectineus	
	Obturator	Adductor brevis	
	Obturator	Adductor longus	
	Obturator	Gracilis	
	Obturator	Adductor magnus	
Sacral plexus L4 to S3	L4, L5, S1	Quadratus femoris	Weakness in extension, adduction, flexion and medial rotation of thigh.
	L4, L5, S1	Gemellus inferior	Weakness in flexion and medial rotation of leg.
	L5, S1, S2	Obturator internus	Weakness in anal sphincter.
	L5, S1, S2	Gemellus superior	Diminished sensation over the posterior thigh, lateral half of the leg and the entire foot
	S1, S2	Piriformis	
	Superior gluteal	Gluteus medius	
	Superior gluteal	Gluteus minimus	
	Superior gluteal	Tensor fasciae latae	
	Inferior gluteal	Gluteus maximus	
	Sciatic	Adductor magnus	
	Sciatic	Semitendinosus	
	Sciatic	Semimembranosus	
	Sciatic	Biceps femoris	

Peripheral nerves	Root	Muscles	Peripheral nerve lesion Signs and symptoms
Femoral	L2, L3	Iliopsoas	Weakness in hip adduction and flexion.
	L2, L3	Sartorius	Weak or absent thigh adduction, flexion and medial rotation.
	L2, L3, L4	Rectus femoris	Weakness or inability to extend the leg at the knee.
	L2, L3, L4	Vastus lateralis	Diminished sensation over the anterior and medial aspect of the thigh and the
	L2, L3, L4	Vastus intermedius	medial aspect of the leg

Table 7.1 Lower extremities (cont'd)

Peripheral nerves	Root	Muscles	Peripheral nerve lesion Signs and symptoms
Obturator	L2, L3, L4 L2, L3	Vastus medialis Pectineus	Weak or absent thigh adduction, flexion, medial and lateral rotation. Diminished sensation over the medial aspect of the thigh
	L2, L3, L4 L2, L3, L4 L2, L3, L4 L2, L3, L4	Adductor brevis Adductor longus Gracilis Adductor magnus	
Superior gluteal	L4, L5, S1 L4, L5, S1 L4, L5, S1	Gluteus medius Gluteus minimus Tensor fasciae latae	Weakness in adduction, flexion and medial rotation of thigh
Inferior gluteal	L5, S1, S2	Gluteus maximus	Weakness in extension, abduction and lateral rotation of thigh
Sciatic	L5, S1, S2 L5, S1, S2 L5, S1, S2 L5, S1, S2 L5, S1, S2	Adductor magnus Semitendinosus Semimembranosus Biceps femoris – long head Short head of biceps femoris	Weakness in extension of the thigh. Weakness in flexion and medial rotation of leg. Diminished sensation over the lateral half of the leg and the entire foot
Deep peroneal	L5, S1 L4, L5 L5, S1 L5, S1 L5, S1	Extensor digitorum longus Tibialis anterior Extensor hallucis longus Peroneus tertius Extensor digitorum	Loss of dorsiflexion (drop foot). Limited inversion/eversion of foot. Unable to extend all toes. Decreased sensation over the dorsum of the foot especially the big toe and the second toe
Superficial peroneal	L5, S1 L5, S1	Peroneus longus Peroneus brevis	Weakness of plantar flexion. Limited eversion of foot. Diminished sensation over the anterolateral part of the leg and the dorsum of the foot

Table 7.1 Lower extremities (cont'd)

Peripheral nerves	Root	Muscles	Peripheral nerve lesion Signs and symptoms
Tibial	S1, S2	Gastrocnemius	Weakness or absent plantar flexion of the foot/toes and flexion of the knee.
	L4, L5, S1	Popliteus	Inability to invert the foot.
	S1, S2	Soleus	Unable to cup sole of foot.
	L5, S1	Tibialis posterior	Sensory problem over the posterior area of the legs.
	L5, S1, S2	Flexor hallucis longus	
	L5, S1, S2	Flexor digitorum longus	
	S1, S2, S3	Abductor digiti minimi	
	S1, S2	Quadratus plantae	
	S1, S2	Flexor digiti minimi	
	S1, S2	Lumbrical	
	S2, S3	Dorsal interossei	
	S2, S3	Plantar interossei	
	S1, S2, S3	Adductor hallucis	
	S1, S2	Abductor hallucis	
	S1, S2	Flexor digitorum brevis	
	S1, S2	Flexor hallucis brevis	

Table 7.2 EMG evaluation

Muscle	Nerves	Roots
Common upper extremity		
– Cervical paraspinal C5	Rami	C5
– Cervical paraspinal C6	Rami	C6
– Cervical paraspinal C7	Rami	C7
– Cervical paraspinal C8	Rami	C8
– Cervical paraspinal T1	Rami	T1
– Deltoid	Axillary	C5–6
– Biceps	Musculocutaneous	C5–6
– Triceps	Radial	C6–7–8
– Pronator teres	Median	C6–7
– Abductor pollicis brevis	Median	C8–T1
– 1st dorsal interosseous	Ulnar	C8–T1
– Abductor digiti minimi	Ulnar	C8–T1
Common lower extremity		
– Lumbar paraspinal L3	Rami	L3
– Lumbar paraspinal L4	Rami	L4
– Lumbar paraspinal L5	Rami	L5
– Lumbar paraspinal S1	Rami	S1
– Gluteus maximus	Inferior gluteal	L5–S2
– Biceps femoris (short head)	Sciatic (peroneal)	L5–S2
– Med gastrocnemius anterior	Tibial	S1–2
tibialis	Deep branch of peroneal	L4–5
– Rectus femoris	Femoral	L2–4
– Biceps femoris (long head)	Sciatic	L5–S2
– Peroneus longus	Superficial branch of peroneal	L5–S1
Other muscles frequently tested		
Forearm		
– Flexor digitorum profundus IV and V	Ulnar	C8, T1
– Flexor pollicis longus	Median (anterior interosseus)	C7–8
– Flexor digitorum superficialis	Median	C7–8
– Flexor carpi radialis	Median	C6–7
– Flexor carpi ulnaris	Ulnar	C7–T1
– Extensor indicis	Radial (posterior interosseus)	C7–8
– Extensor carpi ulnaris	Radial (posterior interosseus)	C7–8
– Extensor carpi radialis	Radial	C6–7
– Extensor digitorum communis	Radial (posterior interosseus)	C7–8
– Brachioradialis	Radial	C5–6
– Anconeus	Radial	C7–8
– Pronator quadratus	Median (anterior interosseus)	C8, T1
Arm		
– Brachialis	Musculocutaneous	C5–6
– Supinator	Radial	C5–6
– Extensor pollicis longus	Radial (posterior interosseus)	C7–8
– Abductor pollicis longus	Radial (posterior interosseus)	C7–8
Shoulder		
– Pectoralis major	Pectoral	C5–T1
– Supraspinatus	Suprascapular	C5–6
– Latissimus dorsi	Thoracodorsal	C6–8
– Teres major	Lower subscapular	C5–6
– Serratus anterior	Long thoracic	C5–7
– Rhomboids	Dorsal scapular	C5
– Levator scapulae	Dorsal scapular	C5
– Infraspinatus	Suprascapular	C5–6
– Trapezius	Spinal accessory	CN XI, C3–4

Table 7.2 EMG evaluation (*cont'd*)

Muscle	Nerves	Roots
Foot		
– Abductor hallucis	Medial plantar	S1–2
– Abductor digiti quinti	Lateral plantar	S1–3
Leg		
– Tibialis posterior	Tibial	L5, S1
– Soleus	Tibial	L5–S2
Thigh		
– Tensor fascia lata	Femoral	L4–5
– Adductor longus	Obturator	L2–4
– Vastus lateralis	Femoral	L2–4
– Vastus medialis	Femoral	L2–4
– Adductor magnus	Obturator, sciatic	L2–S1
– Gracilis	Obturator	L2–4
Hip		
– Gluteus medius	Superior gluteal	L4–S1
– Iliopsoas	Femoral	L2–3
Non-limb		
– Orbicularis oris	Facial	CN VII
– Orbicularis oculi	Facial	CN VII
– Diaphragm	Phrenic	C3–5
– Anal sphincter	Pudendal	S2–4
– Sternocleidomastoid	Spinal accessory	CN XI, C2–3

8

Pitfalls

Lyn Weiss, Jay Weiss, Rebecca Fishman

You've paid attention during EMG lectures and read about EMGs. You feel sufficiently confident to proceed with the study. However, you are not getting the response you were anticipating. What went wrong? Before you start to doubt your abilities, review the pitfalls of EMG testing.

This chapter will emphasize the physiological and human sources of error that can befall both the novice and the experienced electromyographer. These pitfalls are common and straight forward.

Pitfall 1: Not Performing a Good History and Physical Examination

You've heard it before and you'll hear it again. Your history and physical examination are the most important components of an accurate diagnosis – not the EMG. For example, a patient presents to you for electrodiagnostic testing with the diagnosis of carpal tunnel syndrome. On further questioning you discover the patient has neck pain with radiation to the hand and associated paresthesias. You suspect a cervical radiculopathy and examine the patient. He has a positive Spurling's test and upper extremity weakness with a decreased biceps deep tendon reflex. Although the original consultation requested an EMG for carpal tunnel syndrome, your history and physical suggests that you should also test for a possible cervical radiculopathy. This information helps to guide which nerves and muscles you will test during your EMG. Your history and physical, as well as how you interpret your EMG findings, separate you as a physician rather than simply a technician.

Pitfall 2: Technical Factors

Often people assume, when there is an abnormal or unexpected finding, that this represents pathology. Much of the time however, unexpected findings are due to an error by the electromyographer. The main reason for an unobtainable motor or sensory action potential (evoked response) is not stimulating the nerve and/or not recording from the nerve or muscle. This should be addressed methodically. Possible reasons for an unobtainable result are:

- Is a stimulus being delivered? Look for a visible muscle contraction. If there is no muscle contraction:
  a. The stimulator is not working. Try turning down the intensity and stimulating yourself to assess if you feel a shock.
  b. The location is incorrect. Relocate the stimulator.

or

c. The stimulus may not be of a high enough intensity. This may be true especially if there is an excess of adipose tissue. Try increasing the stimulus intensity or duration (pulse width).

● Is the preamplifier on?

Most preamplifiers have a light indicating on/off. If the preamplifier is off, the patient will feel the shock but no response will be recorded.

● Are the settings (gain and sweep) correct?

Attempting to elicit a sensory nerve study at a motor setting will give a flat line because the gain on a motor setting will not be high enough.

● Are wires and electrodes properly connected?

A sine wave usually indicates poor grounding or poor electrode contact.

A large initial positive deflection indicates poor location of electrodes or even reversal of electrodes.

 ## Pitfall 3: Temperature

The temperature of the areas you are testing on your patient can affect the nerve conduction study. You should be aware that *decreasing* limb temperature could affect the latency, amplitude, conduction velocity and duration of sensory nerve action potentials (SNAPs) and compound muscle action potentials (CMAPs) in the following manner:

● Latency   prolonged (0.2 ms/degree centigrade)
● Amplitude   increased with cooling (sensory more than motor)
● Conduction velocity   decreased (1.8 to 2.4 m/s/degree centigrade)
● Duration   increased

You should also be aware that decreased temperature can affect the results of repetitive nerve studies and can cause normal test results in patients with neuromuscular junction disorders.

The limb being tested, ideally, should be continuously monitored for temperature by a temperature probe placed on the limb. When performing nerve conduction studies attempt to maintain the temperature of the upper limbs above 32°C and the lower limbs above 30°C. This can be achieved by warming the area to be tested. It is always better to warm the limb rather than using correcting formulas, as described above (i.e., correct for a temperature of 30°C in the arms by decreasing the latency by 0.4 msec). Tables 8.1 and 8.2 summarize the temperature corrections for nerve conduction studies.

 ## Pitfall 4: Errors in Measurement

In general, the shorter the segment to be measured, the more likely an error in measurement will occur and the more dramatic change there will be in the calculated conduction velocity. For example, a 0.5 cm error in measuring distance will significantly change the conduction velocity if the measured distance is 5 cm (a 10% measurement error). However, if the distance is 10 cm and there is a 0.5 cm error in measurement, this will result in a 5% error. You should try to use segments longer than 10 cm, as there is usually some error when measuring the length of the segment.

Table 8.1 Temperature correction for NCV study. Expected velocity deviation (m/sec) from 32°C

| NCV corrected = factor × (measured skin temperature – 32°C) – NCV measured (m/sec)* | | | | | | |
Measured temperature	Tibial motor	Sural sensory	Peroneal motor	Median motor	Median sensory	Ulnar motor	Ulnar sensory
Factor for NCV change (m/sec/°C)	1.1	1.7	2	1.5	1.4	2.1	1.6
20°C	−13.2	−20.4	−24	−18	−16.8	−25.2	−19.2
21°C	−12.1	−18.7	−22	−16.5	−15.4	−23.1	−17.6
22°C	−11	−17	−20	−15	−14	−21	−16
23°C	−9.9	−15.3	−18	−13.5	−12.6	−18.9	−14.4
24°C	−8.8	−13.6	−16	−12	−11.2	−16.8	−12.8
25°C	−7.7	−11.9	−14	−10.5	−9.8	−14.7	−11.2
26°C	−6.6	−10.2	−12	−9	−8.4	−12.6	−9.6
27°C	−5.5	−8.5	−10	−7.5	−7	−10.5	−8
28°C	−4.4	−6.8	−8	−6	−5.6	−8.4	−6.4
29°C	−3.3	−5.1	−6	−4.5	−4.2	−6.3	−4.8
30°C	−2.2	−3.4	−4	−3	−2.8	−4.2	−3.2
30.5°C	−1.65	−2.55	−3	−2.25	−2.1	−3.15	−2.4
31°C	−1.1	−1.7	−2	−1.5	−1.4	−2.1	−1.6
31.5°C	−0.55	−0.85	−1	−0.75	−0.7	−1.05	−0.8
32°C	0	0	0	0	0	0	0
32.5°C	0.55	0.85	1	0.75	0.7	1.05	0.8
33°C	1.1	1.7	2	1.5	1.4	2.1	1.6
33.5°C	1.65	2.55	3	2.25	2.1	3.15	2.4
34°C	2.2	3.4	4	3	2.8	4.2	3.2
34.5°C	2.75	4.25	5	3.75	3.5	5.25	4
35°C	3.3	5.1	6	4.5	4.2	6.3	4.8
35.5°C	3.85	5.95	7	5.25	4.9	7.35	5.6
36°C	4.4	6.8	8	6	5.6	8.4	6.4

*Delisa J, Lee H, Baran E, Lai K, Spielholz N. Manual of Nerve Conduction Velocity and Clinical Neurophysiology, 3rd Edn. New York: Raven Press, 1994, p. 17–19.

Another source of error in measurement is not measuring over the direct course of the nerve. It is impossible to exactly measure a nerve over the skin. However, measuring over the course of the nerve will minimize the error. This is especially true of the ulnar nerve across the elbow (Fig. 8.1). The ulnar nerve is slack when the elbow is extended, and taut when the elbow is bent. In order to measure the true length of the nerve, the elbow should be flexed to about 70–90 degrees both when the nerve is being stimulated and when the nerve is being measured. Measuring the nerve in the extended elbow position underestimates the true length. This will result in a calculated conduction velocity that is erroneously slow. As all skin measurements are estimates of actual nerve length, the farther the measuring tape is from the actual nerve, the greater the potential for error. Therefore, measurements tend to be less accurate in obese patients.

Table 8.2 Temperature correction for median and ulnar motor/sensory distal latency. Expected latency deviation from 33°C.

Median (or ulnar) motor or sensory NCV or distal latency corrected = −0.2 × (Tst − Tm) + obtained NCV or distal latency.*	
Measured temperature	**−0.2 (Tst − Tm)[†]**
20°C	−2.6
21°C	−2.4
22°C	−2.2
23°C	−2.0
24°C	−1.8
25°C	−1.6
26°C	−1.4
27°C	−1.2
28°C	−1.0
29°C	−0.8
30°C	−0.6
31°C	−0.4
32°C	−0.2
33°C	0.0
34°C	0.2
35°C	0.4
36°C	0.6

*Delisa J, Lee H, Baran E, Lai K, Spielholz N. Manual of Nerve Conduction Velocity and Clinical Neurophysiology, 3rd Edn. New York: Raven Press, 1994, p. 17–19.
[†]Tst = 33°C for wrist. Tm is the measured skin temperature.

Figure 8.1 In order to measure the true length of the ulnar nerve, the elbow should be flexed to about 70–90 degrees both when the nerve is being stimulated and when the nerve is being measured.

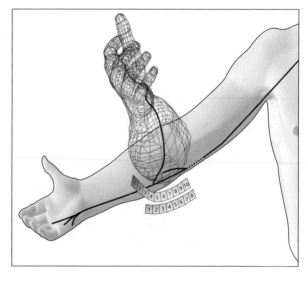

⚠ Pitfall 5: Anomalous Innervation

It is important to remember that human anatomy does not always follow the textbooks and that neurological anomalies exist. There are three anomalous innervations to be especially aware of.

1. Martin–Gruber Anastomosis

This is a *median to ulnar nerve anastomosis* in the forearm (Fig. 8.2). Fibers from the median nerve (usually the anterior interosseus nerve) cross the forearm and travel with the ulnar nerve into the hand. They therefore do not have to traverse the carpal tunnel. This leads to three classic electrodiagnostic findings, which are more pronounced in patients with carpal tunnel syndrome.

a. Positive Deflection of CMAP

The compound muscle action potential (CMAP) will have an initial positive (downward) deflection when stimulating the median nerve at the elbow and picking up over the abductor pollicis brevis (APB) muscle. The reason for this positive deflection is that ulnar fibers traveling with the median nerve stimulate the ulnar intrinsic hand muscles (specifically the adductor pollicis muscle). These fibers arrive at the adductor pollicis muscle before the median fibers arrive at the APB muscle, since they are not delayed across the carpal tunnel as the median fibers are. Since the motor point of the adductor muscle is not over the recording electrode, a positive deflection will occur.

b. Increased Conduction Velocity or Negative Conduction Velocity

The median nerve is usually slowed somewhat as it traverses the carpal tunnel. (This is why the latency for the median nerve at the wrist is usually more than the ulnar nerve at the wrist.) If a Martin–Gruber anastomosis exists, proximal stimulation will result in a 'normal' latency because the fastest fibers (those upon which the latency is based) are actually ulnar fibers that do not have to travel through the carpal tunnel. The calculated conduction velocity is therefore based on a proximal stimulation (which will be falsely

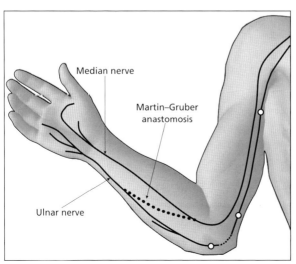

Figure 8.2
Martin–Gruber anastomosis.

Median nerve

Martin–Gruber anastomosis

Ulnar nerve

shortened by picking up over the ulnarly innervated adductor pollicis muscle) and the distal stimulation (picking up over the median innervated APB muscle). With carpal tunnel syndrome, the difference in these latencies will be exaggerated, and may actually lead to a negative conduction velocity (where the elbow latency is less than the wrist latency).

c. CMAP Amplitude Changes

With a Martin–Gruber anastomosis, the proximal CMAP amplitude will be larger than the distal amplitude (when stimulating the median nerve and picking up over the APB). This is because at the elbow, in addition to median fibers destined for the APB, ulnar fibers destined for the adductor pollicis muscle are stimulated. (These fibers will be traveling with the ulnar nerve because of the anastomosis). Since the adductor pollicis muscle is close to the APB, the two CMAPs summate to give the appearance of a larger amplitude CMAP with proximal stimulation. (Remember that this 'larger amplitude' actually includes the response from the stimulated adductor muscle – an ulnarly innervated muscle that is not usually activated with pure median nerve stimulation.) For the same reason, this can also give larger amplitude on ulnar nerve studies when stimulating the ulnar nerve at the wrist rather than at the elbow. The lost fibers in the elbow amplitude can be 'found' with median stimulation at the elbow.

2. Riche–Cannieu Anastomosis

This is a communication between the *deep branch* of the *ulnar nerve* and the *recurrent branch* of the *median nerve* in the hand. With this anastomosis, the ulnar nerve may innervate the thenar muscles along with the median nerve.

If a patient with Riche–Cannieu anastomosis had a complete laceration of the median nerve at the wrist; he or she may still retain thenar muscle function, as some of these muscles may be innervated by the ulnar nerve (via the anastomosis). On EMG evaluation, a median nerve injury at the wrist, which should result in fibrillation potentials and positive sharp waves in median innervated hand muscles, may result in a normal study. Conversely, an ulnar nerve lesion at the elbow may result in spontaneous activity in median innervated hand muscles.

3. Accessory Peroneal Nerve (Fig. 8.3)

The *accessory deep peroneal nerve* is a branch from the *superficial peroneal nerve* that travels posterior to the lateral malleolus and can innervate the lateral portion of the extensor digitorum brevis (EDB) muscle. Therefore a patient may have a peroneal nerve injury with loss of muscle function while still maintaining EDB function. This anomaly is usually picked up when the amplitude of the peroneal CMAP is larger on proximal (fibular head) stimulation than on distal (ankle) stimulation. This results because fibers from the accessory branch (posterior to the lateral malleolus) are not activated with ankle stimulation but are activated with fibular head stimulation. Usually, stimulation posterior to the lateral malleolus (with pickup over the extensor digitorum brevis) will produce a waveform that (in amplitude) along with the ankle stimulation summates to the amplitude of the proximal (fibular head) stimulation (Fig. 8.4):

Accessory peroneal nerve amplitude (posterior to lateral malleolus) +
ankle peroneal amplitude = fibular head amplitude

 ## Pitfall 6: Stimulating Over Subcutaneous or Adipose Tissue

While performing NCS, you must be aware that placing the stimulator over areas of increased adipose or subcutaneous tissue can cause submaximal stimulation. This may

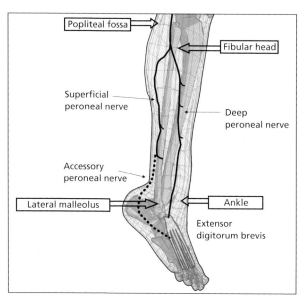

Figure 8.3
Accessory peroneal nerve.

Popliteal fossa

Fibular head

Superficial peroneal nerve

Deep peroneal nerve

Accessory peroneal nerve

Lateral malleolus

Ankle

Extensor digitorum brevis

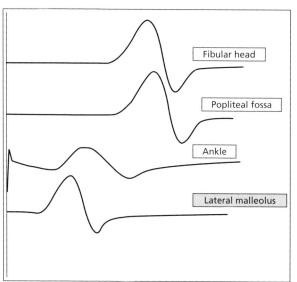

Figure 8.4
Stimulation posterior to the lateral malleolus (with pickup over the extensor digitorum brevis) will produce a waveform that (in amplitude) along with the ankle stimulation summates to the amplitude of the proximal (fibular head) stimulation.

Fibular head

Popliteal fossa

Ankle

Lateral malleolus

result in decreased amplitude of the CMAP. To correct this, press deeply with the stimulator until the desired results are obtained. You can also increase the pulse width. Care must be taken so as not to stimulate a different nerve located nearby.

Pitfall 7: Anatomy Error

Obviously, if you are stimulating or placing a needle in the incorrect nerve or muscle, your results will be inaccurate. To help identify the correct muscles have the patient activate the muscle first and palpate for correct placement.

Pitfall 8: Physiologic Factors

Human physiology presents various factors that can significantly affect NCS. To professionally and appropriately conduct EMG examinations the relevant factors must be considered.

Age

Age affects electrodiagnostic studies in both the very young and the very old patient. The effect of age is most significant from birth to one year when myelination is incomplete. In the newborn, nerve conduction velocities are approximately 50% of adult values.[1] By one year of age the velocities reach 75% and by 3–5 years myelination is complete and children's values can be compared to adult normative data.

In adults, NCS values also change as people age. Typically, the older you get, the slower your nerves will conduct. Although these changes are fairly insignificant in the middle-aged adult, they do become more pronounced in the older adult. For example, a median motor conduction velocity of 46 meters/second in a 90-year-old patient would be normal even though generally the lower limit of normal is 50 meters/second.[2] The usual corrective factor is about one to two meters/second slowing per decade of life after age 60.[3]

In NCS, the amplitude of the SNAP and CMAP may also be affected by age. It is estimated that the SNAP amplitude may decrease by as much as 50% in a 70-year-old patient. This means that very low or even absent sensory nerve responses in the elderly should be interpreted with caution, as they may be normal given the patient's advanced age. It is important to review the entire study, including the different technical factors that may affect the results, before arriving at a conclusion.

In the elderly, when dropout of motor units occurs due to normal aging, the body compensates with axonal sprouting leading to reinnervation. These reinnervated fibers are more likely to fire asynchronously. Therefore, during the EMG portion of the test, in the older adult, the MUAP duration may *increase* with age. In childhood, the MUAP duration increases due to physiologic growth of the muscle fiber and motor unit size.

In summary, age affects NCS in babies with marked slowing of the velocities, due to incomplete myelination. In the elderly, NCS are slower with reduced amplitudes and EMG findings reveal increased duration of the MUAP.

Height

If you can remember that nerve conduction studies are normally faster in the arms than in the legs, then the effect of height will make sense to you. Basically, the longer the extremity, the slower the nerves conduct. So, in the arms they conduct more quickly and in shorter people they conduct more quickly. This is probably due to the fact that there is distal tapering of the nerve. The longer the limb, the more tapering and therefore, the slower the conduction velocity will be. Also, longer limbs are probably cooler and this too will slow the conduction velocity.

Weight

Weight is not a well-appreciated physiologic factor. However, in obese individuals, it may be difficult to stimulate the nerve directly. Additional stimulus intensity or duration may be required. This is due to the electrical stimulation having to pass through additional adipose tissue before reaching the nerve. During the EMG portion of the test, technical difficulties may arise when the needle is not long enough to be easily inserted into the muscle.

Pitfall 9: Non-physiologic Factors (Machine or Environmentally Related)

Noise

Noise is exactly what it says – noise. Noise is any electrical signal that is not the desired biological signal you are studying. When you have a lot of noise, it is difficult to hear what you need to hear (and to see what you need to see on the screen). Electrical noise is present to some degree in all electrodiagnostic labs. The most frequent form of noise is 60 Hz interference, which is due to ubiquitous electrical appliances (e.g., lights, computers, fans and heaters). In order to minimize noise, check all of your equipment:

- Wires should be intact (not frayed or damaged).
- Electrodes, including the ground, should be securely attached.
- The ground should be between the recording and stimulating electrodes.
- The skin should be properly cleaned (usually with alcohol).
- Electrode gel needs to be applied.
- The closer the electrodes are to each other, the less likely there will be noise.
- Unplug equipment (e.g., exam tables) that you are not using while performing the study.
- Turning off fluorescent lights will cut down on the interference from unwanted signals.

Many EMG machines have a 60-cycle notch filter that will filter out only electrical response firing at 60 Hz. This can be beneficial in eliminating 60 Hz interference. One theoretical downside is you can eliminate a potential whose frequency is 60 cycles, i.e. a fib or positive sharp wave that is firing at 60 Hz.

In summary, there are a number of factors that may result in an abnormal finding. Before you decide that this is true pathology you must consider the possible pitfalls discussed in this chapter.

- Remember to do a thorough history and physical examination.
- Know your anatomy.
- Be aware of anomalous innervations and temperature changes.
- Keep the limb appropriately warm
- Measure correctly.
- If abnormalities are encountered – check and recheck your stimulating electrodes, wires and placement.

REFERENCES

1. Preston DC, Shapiro BE. Electromyography and Neuromuscular Disorders. Newton, Massachusetts: Butterworth-Heinemann, 1998, p. 86.
2. Preston DC, Shapiro BE. Electromyography and Neuromuscular Disorders. Newton, Massachusetts: Butterworth-Heinemann, 1998, p. 87.
3. Dumitru D. Electrodiagnostic Medicine. Philadelphia, PA: Hanley & Belfus, Inc., 1995, p. 39.

9

Carpal Tunnel Syndrome

Lyn Weiss

Carpal tunnel syndrome (symptomatic median neuropathy at the wrist) is the most common focal nerve entrapment, and a frequent reason for electrodiagnostic consultation. Electrodiagnostic testing is the *only* available method to assess the physiologic changes that occur in carpal tunnel syndrome.

 ## Clinical Presentation

Classic symptoms of carpal tunnel syndrome (CTS) include paresthesias and numbness in the thumb, index and long fingers, and radial half of the ring finger (Fig. 9.1). Pain in the hand may also be present, and radiation proximally is not uncommon. The symptoms are frequently more prominent at night. The patient may complain of an inability to perform fine motor tasks and/or weakness of the hand. Certain medical and/or physical conditions predispose patients to CTS. These include diabetes, pregnancy, thyroid disorders, repetitive strain, rheumatoid arthritis, gout, peripheral neuropathy, and edema. A good history is therefore important.

On physical examination, there may be a sensory deficit in the radial three and a half digits. Weakness of pinch strength may also be noted. In severe cases of carpal tunnel syndrome, wasting of the thenar eminence may be present. Provocative tests may reproduce the symptoms. These include *Tinel's test* (percussion of the median nerve about the wrist) and *Phalen's test* (maximum flexion of the wrist, which is maintained for one to two minutes). Since CTS can be confused with other disorders, a thorough physical examination is always important.

 ## Anatomy

The carpal tunnel is a fixed space that includes nine tendons (four flexor digitorum superficialis tendons, four flexor digitorum profundus tendons, and the flexor pollicis

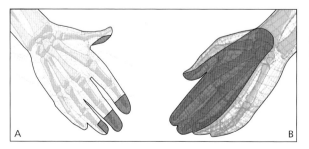

Figure 9.1
Median nerve sensory distribution (A), palmar (B).

Figure 9.2
Anatomy of the
carpal tunnel.

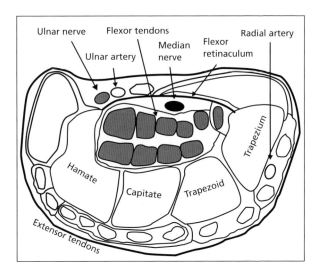

longus tendon), and the median nerve (Fig. 9.2). The carpal tunnel is bound dorsally by the carpal bones and volarly by the transverse carpal ligament (flexor retinaculum). When the space in the tunnel becomes restricted, the median nerve can become compressed.

 Electrodiagnostic Findings

In order to do a complete electrodiagnostic assessment of the median nerve, the affected extremity must be compared to the unaffected side and to another nerve in the same hand, usually the ulnar nerve. Sensory and motor studies should be performed, as well as needle testing. When performing nerve conduction studies, it is imperative that the distance from the active electrode to the stimulation site be recorded. If a person has a large hand, and the distance for the distal latency for motor nerve conduction studies is not the standard 8 cm, an increased latency will have no real meaning (Fig. 9.3).

Sensory Nerve Conduction Studies

Sensory nerve action potentials (SNAPs) are usually the first potentials affected in carpal tunnel syndrome. A useful technique is to compare SNAPs recorded at mid palm and across the carpal tunnel. Usually, a distance of 7 cm from the ring electrode on the second digit to mid palm and then another 7 cm to the carpal tunnel (14 cm total) is used. However, since it is important to stimulate *across* the carpal tunnel, a larger distance can be used and recorded. Although every lab has its own standards of normal, *in general* a velocity of less than 44 meters/second across the carpal tunnel indicates slowing.

Normal mid palm SNAPs confirm that the slowing is only across the carpal tunnel, although in moderate or severe cases, Wallerian degeneration may occur and affect these distal SNAPs as well. Median SNAPs may also be compared to ulnar SNAPs on the same finger. A greater than 0.5 milliseconds difference between the two sensory latencies indicates CTS. Decreased amplitude on the affected side could indicate either an axonal lesion of the median nerve (not specific as to where along the course of the nerve) or a conduction block across the carpal tunnel (if proximal amplitude is less than 50% of

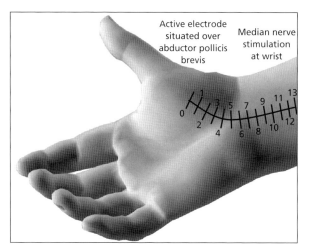

Figure 9.3
Distance from the active electrode to the stimulation site for *motor* nerve conduction studies. Note that in a large hand, the distance from the APB to the wrist may be more than 8 cm. The latency will be longer if the distance is greater.

Within the figure: Active electrode situated over abductor pollicis brevis · Median nerve stimulation at wrist

distal mid palm amplitude). An amplitude difference of more than 50% (as compared to the median sensory amplitude on the non-affected side) is considered significant.

Motor Nerve Conduction Studies

The distal latency of the compound muscle action potential (CMAP) is an important parameter in assessing for motor fiber involvement in CTS. As in sensory studies, the distance from the active electrode to the stimulation site must be standardized. Many laboratories use a distance of 8 cm. With this distance, a latency of more than 4.2 milliseconds usually indicates CTS. The ulnar nerve must also be assessed to ensure that there is not a generalized motor neuropathy present. A median to ulnar distal latency difference of more than 1 millisecond also indicates CTS, as with sensory conduction studies. Decreased amplitude on the affected side could indicate either an axonal lesion of the median nerve (not specific as to where along the nerve) or a conduction block across the carpal tunnel.

Late Responses

Late responses (F-waves and H-reflexes) are generally not helpful in the evaluation of CTS because they are non-specific and the area of greatest interest is not being assessed directly. The areas of interest are easily directly assessed by conventional motor and sensory studies.

EMG

EMG testing should be performed to provide evidence of axonal damage (fibrillation potentials or positive sharp waves), and/or reinnervation. Testing should include the abductor pollicis brevis (APB) muscle. If spontaneous activity is present in this muscle, other muscles should be tested to ensure that the diagnosis is indeed CTS, as CTS can coexist with other conditions. Specifically, a more proximal median muscle should be tested to be sure there is not a median neuropathy elsewhere along the nerve's course. In addition, a non-median innervated C8 muscle should be tested. Finally, especially if there is any indication of a neck problem, the cervical paraspinal muscles may be tested

Table 9.1 Median nerve innervated muscles and expected electromyography changes for focal median nerve injuries

Muscles innervated by median nerve from proximal to distal	Nerve	Muscles affected in the ligament of Struther's syndrome	Muscles affected in pronator teres syndrome	Muscles affected in anterior interosseous nerve (AIN) syndrome	Muscles affected in carpal tunnel syndrome
Pronator teres (forearm)	Median nerve	✓			
Flexor carpi radialis	Median nerve	✓	✓		
Palmaris longus	Median nerve	✓	✓		
Flexor digitorum superficialis	Median nerve	✓	✓		
Flexor digitorum profundus (digits 2 and 3)	AIN	✓	✓	✓	
Flexor pollicis longus	AIN	✓	✓	✓	
Pronator quadratus	AIN	✓	✓	✓	
Abductor pollicis brevis (distal to wrist)	Median nerve	✓	✓		✓
Opponens pollicis	Median nerve	✓	✓		✓
Flexor pollicis brevis (superficial head)	Median nerve	✓	✓		✓
1st, 2nd lumbrical	Median nerve	✓	✓		✓
Clinical sign: Nocturnal paresthesia		Yes	Yes	No	Yes
Pain in the palm and thenar eminence		Yes	Yes, plus pain in elbow region	No, but pain in volar wrist or forearm	Yes
Difficult to form 'O' sign		Yes	Yes	Yes	No
Weakness of pronation		Yes*	No	No	No
Abnormal sensation in palm		Yes†	Yes†	No	No
NCV Conduction block		Upper arm to elbow segment	Elbow to wrist segment	No conduction block	Across wrist

*Weakness of pronation differentiates ligament of Struther's syndrome from pronator teres syndrome.
†The palmar cutaneous branch is spared in carpal tunnel syndrome because it passes superficial to the carpal tunnel. Sensory deficits in the palm and thenar eminence can help to differentiate pronator teres syndrome or ligament of Struther's syndrome from carpal tunnel syndrome.

to rule out a cervical radiculopathy. If there is conduction block in the median nerve, recruitment may be decreased in the APB without evidence of spontaneous potentials.

 ## Written Report

The written conclusion should include the following:

1. Whether or not carpal tunnel syndrome is present electrodiagnostically.
2. The severity of the CTS (mild, moderate or severe).[1] As a general guideline:
   a. *Mild* – median sensory nerve conduction slowing and/or median sensory amplitude decreased but more than 50% of reference value (no motor involvement).
   b. *Moderate* – Median sensory and motor slowing, *and/or* SNAP amplitude less than 50% of the reference value.
   c. *Severe* – Absence of median SNAP with motor slowing *or* median motor slowing with decreased median motor amplitude *or* CMAP abnormalities with evidence of axonal injury on needle testing of the thenar muscles.
3. Whether sensory and/or motor fibers are affected.
4. If spontaneous activity is noted in the abductor pollicis brevis (fibrillation potentials and/or positive sharp waves).

 ## Summary

The classic electrodiagnostic findings in carpal tunnel syndrome may include:

1. slowing of median sensory nerve conduction velocity across the carpal tunnel
2. prolonged distal latency of the median motor nerve
3. low amplitude of the median SNAP
4. low amplitude of the median CMAP
5. spontaneous potentials (fibs and/or PSWs) in the abductor pollicis brevis muscle.

For a summary of NCS/EMG findings in median neuropathy, see Table 9.1.

REFERENCE

1. O'Young B, Young M, Stiens S. PM&R Secrets. Philadelphia, PA: Hanley & Belfus, Inc., 1997, p. 188.

10

Ulnar Neuropathy

Lyn Weiss

 ## Clinical Presentation

Ulnar neuropathy is the second most frequent entrapment neuropathy of the upper extremity (carpal tunnel syndrome being the most common). The ulnar nerve can be compressed at several locations along its course. Most commonly, compression occurs in its superficial location at the *elbow*. Often this occurs when someone leans on his or her elbow (e.g., at a desk at work) or when the elbow is repetitively flexed and extended (e.g., carpenter or assembly worker). Scarring of the ulnar collateral ligament, arthritis within the ulnar groove, traction at a compression site or valgus overload in throwing athletes may all contribute to the injury. Patients typically report paresthesias, pain and numbness in the little and ring fingers, which can worsen with elbow flexion. Pain may be experienced throughout the arm (Fig. 10.1).

Ulnar neuropathy at the *wrist* is less common and occurs in a canal formed by the hamate and its hook and the pisiform. These are connected by an aponeurosis, which forms the roof of *Guyon's canal*. This canal contains the ulnar artery, vein and nerve. People who put a lot of pressure on their wrists, particularly in extension (e.g., cyclists and cane users) are at risk for this injury.

On physical examination in patients with ulnar neuropathy at the elbow, the ulnar nerve may be palpable in the post-condylar groove, especially with elbow flexion. There may be a sensory deficit in the fifth digit and the ulnar half of the fourth digit. Any altered sensation should be distal to the wrist, as the *medial antebrachial cutaneous nerve* supplies sensation above the wrist. An important clinical clue as to whether an ulnar lesion is at the elbow or the wrist is assessment of the dorsal ulnar cutaneous branch of the ulnar nerve. This nerve usually branches before the wrist so it is spared in ulnar nerve lesions at the wrist. This nerve provides sensation to the dorsal lateral aspect of the hand. With ulnar neuropathy at either the wrist or elbow, hand intrinsic muscle weakness may be evident, and in severe cases clawing of the fourth and fifth digits (with attempted hand opening) and atrophy of the intrinsic muscles (particularly the first dorsal interosseous muscle) may be obvious (Fig. 10.2).

Wartenberg's sign (abduction of the 4th and 5th digits) may occur, especially if the patient is asked to put his or her hands in the pants' pocket. *Froment's sign* may also be present. This is seen when a patient is asked to grasp a piece of paper between the thumb and radial side of the second digit. When the examiner tries to pull the paper out of the patient's hand, the patient will use the flexor pollicis longus muscle (innervated by the intact median nerve) to substitute for the adductor pollicis muscle (innervated by the affected ulnar nerve) (Fig. 10.3).

Figure 10.1
(A) Ulnar nerve:
cutaneous
distribution.
(B) Detail of
hand.

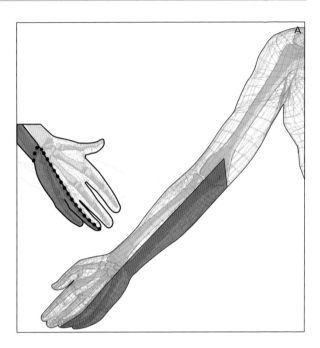

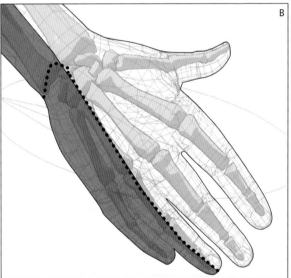

On physical examination of ulnar neuropathy at the wrist there are three basic types of lesions that can occur which affect the presentation significantly.

Type I affects the trunk of the ulnar nerve proximally in Guyon's canal and typically involves both the motor and the sensory fibers. This means that clinically the patient presents with numbness, pain, paresthesias and weakness in an ulnar distribution. There

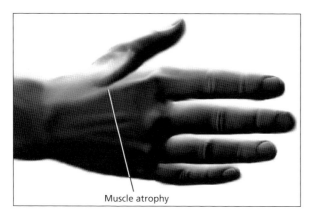

Figure 10.2
Atrophy of the intrinsic muscles – particularly the first dorsal interosseous muscle.

Muscle atrophy

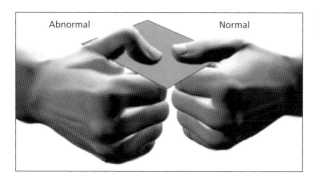

Abnormal   Normal

Figure 10.3
Froment's sign.

may be a notable sensory loss and the hand intrinsic muscles may show wasting in severe cases.

In *Type II* only the deep motor branch is affected distally in Guyon's canal. Sensation is typically spared and the abductor digiti quinti as well as the hypothenar muscles may or may not be spared.

In *Type III* only the superficial branch of the ulnar nerve is affected. The superficial branch provides sensation to the volar aspect of the fourth and fifth fingers and the hypothenar eminence. Strength is generally preserved throughout, as is sensation of the dorsal aspect of the hand.

 ## Anatomy

Anatomy of the ulnar nerve renders it vulnerable to compression at two main locations – the elbow and the wrist (Fig. 10.4).

At the elbow (the most common site for ulnar nerve compression), the ulnar nerve is relatively superficial. The nerve can be compromised by pressure (such as repetitive leaning on the elbow), bony deformity (such as tardy ulnar palsy – ulnar neuropathy after a distal humeral fracture with development of a cubital valgus deformity), chronic subluxation, or in the cubital tunnel.

Figure 10.4
Anatomy of the
ulnar nerve.

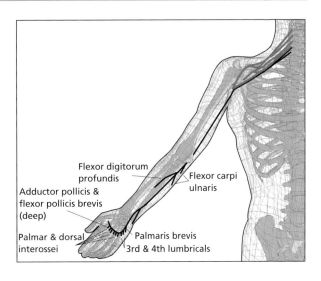

Cubital tunnel syndrome is compression of the ulnar nerve at or beneath the proximal edge of the flexor carpi ulnaris aponeurosis and the arcuate ligament (also referred to as the humeroulnar arcade – HUA). With elbow flexion, the distance between the olecranon process and the medial epicondyle decreases. Elbow flexion stretches and tightens the arcuate ligament, which can compress the ulnar nerve. The volume of the cubital tunnel is maximal in extension, and can decrease by 50% with elbow flexion.

The ulnar nerve is also vulnerable to compression at *Guyon's canal*. This is a fibro-osseous compartment in the wrist where the ulnar nerve is bound by the transverse carpal ligament, the volar carpal ligament, the pisiform bone and the hook of the hamate. When compression occurs at Guyon's canal, the superficial and the deep branches of the ulnar nerve may be affected, but again, the dorsal ulnar cutaneous nerve would not be affected.

 ## Electrodiagnostic Findings

Electrodiagnostic testing of the ulnar nerve can help to establish the existence of a lesion, localize the injury, prognosticate, and exclude other conditions that may mimic an ulnar neuropathy. In severe cases of ulnar neuropathy, when surgery is being considered, electrodiagnostic testing can direct the surgeon to the area of entrapment. Moreover, C8 radiculopathy can present with symptoms similar to an ulnar neuropathy, and electrodiagnostic testing can help differentiate the two conditions.

While different causes of ulnar neuropathy at the elbow may benefit from different surgical procedures, electrodiagnostic studies cannot reliably and consistently differentiate between tardy ulnar palsy, retrocondylar compression and cubital tunnel entrapment. Nevertheless, these studies can be very helpful in distinguishing ulnar neuropathy at the elbow from other pathology.

Sensory Nerve Conduction Studies

Sensory nerve action potentials (SNAPs) can be affected in ulnar neuropathy since the lesion is distal to the dorsal root ganglion (see Chapter 12, Radiculopathy). This is in contrast to a C8 radiculopathy, where the lesion is proximal to the dorsal root ganglion and the SNAPs are not affected. If an ulnar lesion affects the sensory fibers, SNAP amplitudes will usually be reduced. A side-to-side difference of more than 50% is significant for sensory axonal loss. It should be noted that a Type II lesion at the wrist, as described above, would affect the ulnar nerve, but spare the sensory fibers.

In an ulnar neuropathy, it is important to test not only the SNAP to the 5th digit, but also the dorsal ulnar cutaneous nerve. This sensory branch of the ulnar nerve is given off 5–10 cm proximal to the wrist and supplies sensation to the dorsum of the 5th and ulnar side of the 4th digit. A lesion distal to the branching of the dorsal ulnar cutaneous nerve (e.g., at the wrist) should yield a normal dorsal ulnar cutaneous response, but an abnormal ulnar sensory response to the 5th digit. By contrast, an ulnar neuropathy at the elbow would affect both the dorsal ulnar cutaneous response and the ulnar sensory response to the 5th digit.

Motor Nerve Conduction Studies

Slowing of latency and/or conduction velocity can indicate a demyelinating process in the ulnar nerve. In general, a prolonged distal latency of the compound muscle action potential (CMAP) indicates slowing of the ulnar nerve across the wrist, provided there are no other indications of a generalized condition (i.e., the median distal motor latency is normal and conduction throughout the rest of the ulnar nerve is normal). Slowing of the ulnar nerve across the elbow is quite common. Slowing of proximal conduction velocity of more than 10 meters/second is considered significant (compared to the distal conduction velocity on the same side).

Assessment of amplitude can be tricky, especially if a conduction block is present. Low CMAP amplitude throughout the nerve indicates an axonal lesion. However, an amplitude drop when stimulating over a portion of a nerve indicates a conduction block. (Provided there is no anomalous innervation, and ample stimulation is applied directly over the nerve.) A drop in amplitude from the distal to the proximal site of more than 20–30% usually indicates either a conduction block or a Martin–Gruber anastomosis. Evaluating the median nerve CMAP morphology can check for the presence of a Martin–Gruber anastomosis (see Chapter 8, Pitfalls).

When performing nerve conduction studies of the ulnar nerve, position and measurement across the elbow is very important. The elbow should be held in a *flexed* position of 70–90 degrees. The main reasons for this are:

1. The ulnar nerve is redundant in the extended position. Therefore, measurement in extension does not measure the nerve's true anatomical length. The conduction velocity will be falsely slowed since the distance will be under-estimated and the numerator will be decreased in the equation for velocity:

$$velocity = distance / time$$

2. Maintaining the elbow in a flexed position is more likely to reproduce the symptoms of ulnar entrapment at the elbow, if it exists.

If an ulnar neuropathy is expected from the patient's clinical presentation, but the CMAPs are normal, consider using the first dorsal interosseus (FDI) muscle for the active electrode instead of the abductor digiti quinti. In some patients, the FDI is more affected, and therefore more likely to yield a positive result.

Inching is a useful technique for localizing entrapment along the course of a nerve (Fig. 10.5). It is particularly useful in ulnar neuropathy across the elbow when surgery is being considered, as it localizes entrapment more precisely than conventional studies.

Figure 10.5
Inching technique for ulnar nerve.

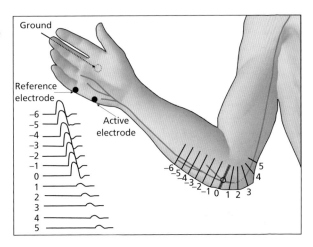

With the elbow flexed, segments of 1 cm are marked on the patient's skin both proximal and distal to the elbow. The ulnar nerve is then stimulated at 1 cm intervals, and the resulting CMAPs compared. An increase in latency of ≥ 0.4 milliseconds/cm is indicative of focal slowing. A substantial amplitude drop from one segment to a more proximal segment indicates a conduction block across that area. One must interpret these results with caution, as the margin of error is high with a small distance. Therefore, an amplitude change is much more significant than a latency change.

When performing nerve conduction studies across the elbow, a distance of at least 10 cm should be used in order to decrease the margin of error.

Late Responses

Late responses (F-waves and H-reflexes) are generally not helpful in the evaluation of an ulnar neuropathy, because they are non-specific.

EMG

EMG testing in cases of ulnar neuropathy can be difficult to interpret because of the muscles innervated by the ulnar nerve and their location. The abductor digiti minimi (ADM) (sometimes referred to as the abductor digiti quinti – ADQ) and the first dorsal interosseous (FDI) are the most commonly tested ulnar innervated hand muscles. If there is an axonotmetic lesion, these are more likely to be positive than the forearm muscles. The flexor carpi ulnaris (FCU) and FDP IV/V are the only ulnar proximal muscles to the wrist. However, in ulnar nerve lesions at the elbow, the FCP and FDP muscles are usually spared. This may be due to:

1. the FCU and FDP receiving their innervation proximal to the medical epicondyle or
2. the fibers to the FCU being situated more medially and therefore are more protected.

Consequently, if the needle examination of the FCU and FDP is negative, an ulnar nerve lesion proximal to the wrist cannot be ruled out. For this reason, frequently the conduction studies are the most important tests in localizing an ulnar lesion.

If an axonal lesion is present anywhere along the course of the nerve, spontaneous activity (fibrillation potentials and positive sharp waves) may be present in muscles distal to the lesion.

Table 10.1 Ulnarly innervated muscles and electromyography for the focal ulnar nerve injury

Location	Muscles innervated by ulnar nerve from proximal to distal upper extremity	Innervated nerve	Neurogenic change in muscles in ulnar entrapment injury at arm (retrocondylar groove)	Neurogenic change in muscles in ulnar entrapment at elbow (cubital tunnel syndrome)	Neurogenic change in muscles in ulnar entrapment at wrist (Guyon's canal)*
Forearm	Flexor carpi ulnaris	Ulnar	✓	✓	
	Flexor digitorum profundus (to digits 4 and 5)	Ulnar	✓	✓	
Hand	Palmaris brevis	Ulnar	✓	✓	
	Abductor digiti minimi	Ulnar	✓	✓	✓
	Opponens digiti minimi	Ulnar	✓	✓	✓
	Flexor digiti minimi	Ulnar	✓	✓	✓
	Palmar interosseous	Ulnar	✓	✓	✓
	Dorsal interosseous (the first one)	Ulnar	✓	✓	✓
	Adductor pollicis	Ulnar	✓	✓	✓
	Lumbricals (two medial ones)	Ulnar	✓	✓	✓
Clinical sign	Paresthesia, pain, or numbness from 4th and 5th digits and hypothenar eminence		Up to the elbow, exacerbated by prolonged elbow flexion	Up to (or slightly distal to) the elbow, exacerbated by prolonged elbow flexion	Volar aspect only of digits 4 and 5
	Loss of sensation over the ulnar dorsal surface of the hand		Yes	Yes	No
	Claw hand			May occur	May occur
	Weakness of the flexor carpi ulnaris and flexor digitorum profundus (digits 4 and 5)		May occur	Variable	No
	Weakness of first dorsal interosseous muscle: Froment's sign		Yes	May occur	May occur

*In or about Guyon's canal the ulnar nerve divides into a superficial and deep branch. The superficial branch of the ulnar nerve innervates the palmaris brevis muscle. The deep branch of the ulnar nerve travels between the abductor digiti minimi and flexor digiti minimi muscles.

Summary

In summary, the classic electrodiagnostic findings in ulnar neuropathy at the elbow may include:

1. slowing of the ulnar motor nerve conduction velocity across the elbow
2. decreased amplitude of the ulnar motor CMAP with stimulation above the elbow (conduction block)
3. decreased amplitude of the ulnar SNAP
4. spontaneous potentials (fibs and PSWs) in ulnarly innervated muscles
5. decreased amplitude of the dorsal ulnar cutaneous SNAP.

See Table 10.1 for a summary of electrodiagnostic findings in ulnar neuropathy.

11

Radial Neuropathy

Julie Silver

Clinical Presentation

As with any nerve, the radial nerve is at risk for injury in a number of locations and from a number of factors, including trauma such as a humeral fracture or compression due to an extrinsic force. The most common sites of injury are at the spiral groove (honeymooner's palsy or Saturday night palsy) and in the forearm where the nerve penetrates the supinator muscle. Less common sites include the axilla (due to crutches), elbow (in radius dislocation injuries) and the wrist (due to handcuffs). The recurrent epicondylar branch may be associated with tennis elbow. If only the posterior interosseous nerve is affected, patients will complain of weakness without sensory symptoms. Injury to the antebrachial cutaneous nerve or the superficial radial sensory nerve (e.g., from lacerations at the wrist or even a watchband that is too tight) can cause numbness and paresthesias in a radial distribution (Fig. 11.1). There may or may not be associated pain. When pain is present, it can mimic or be associated with tenosynovitis (e.g., De Quervain's syndrome) of the thumb.

The physical examination is consistent with sensory and strength deficits that are in the distribution of the radial nerve or one of its branches. It is important to know the anatomy of the radial nerve in order to perform a competent physical examination. Usually the most obvious physical deficit is wrist drop.

Anatomy

The radial nerve branches from the posterior cord of the brachial plexus (Fig. 11.2) and in the proximal arm gives off the following sensory branches:

1. posterior cutaneous nerve of the arm
2. lower lateral cutaneous nerve of the arm and
3. posterior cutaneous nerve of the forearm.

Also in the proximal arm, the radial nerve supplies motor branches to the triceps and anconeus. The radial nerve then wraps around the humerus in the *spiral groove* (one of the most common sites of injury) and supplies motor branches to the brachioradialis, the long head of the extensor carpi radialis and the supinator. Just distal to the lateral epicondyle, the radial nerve splits into the posterior interosseous nerve (motor) and the superficial radial sensory nerve (sensory). The superficial radial sensory nerve supplies the lateral dorsum of the hand. The posterior interosseous nerve enters the supinator muscle under the arcade of Frohse (another common site of compression) and supplies motor nerves to the wrist, thumb and finger extensors.

Figure 11.1
Radial nerve –
cutaneous
distribution.

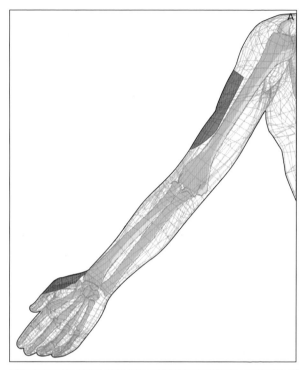

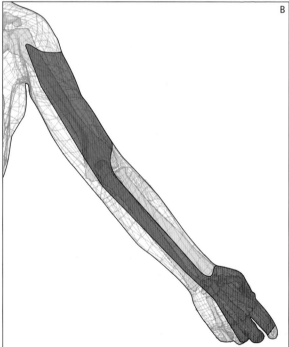

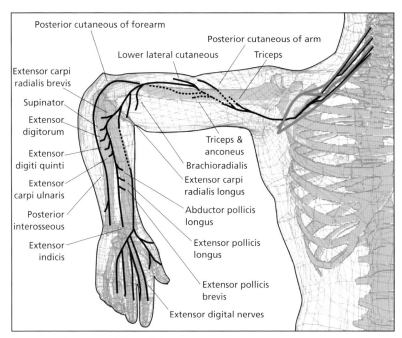

Figure 11.2 Branches of the radial nerve.

Radial nerve injuries can be classified into injuries:

- around the axilla
- associated with the spiral groove
- of the posterior interosseous nerve or
- of the superficial radial sensory nerves.

It may also help to remember that the radial nerve is responsible for the so-called *Saturday night palsy* which is classically compression of the radial nerve when someone who perhaps is very fatigued or intoxicated lies with the arm draped over the back of a chair or some other fixed object.

 ## Electrodiagnostic Findings

Sensory Nerve Conduction Studies

If the superficial radial sensory nerve is affected, in demyelinating lesions there will be a prolonged distal latency if the lesion is distal to the site of stimulation. In axonal lesions there will be reduced amplitude of the sensory nerve action potential (SNAP) regardless of the location of the lesion (as long as it is distal to the dorsal root ganglion). In cases where the SNAP is normal but the patient clinically has a radial sensory deficit, this may be because: the study was done too early (it takes 4–7 days for Wallerian degeneration to occur); the lesion may be proximal to the dorsal root ganglion (i.e., root level); or the lesion may be proximal to the site of stimulation.

Table 11.1 Radial nerve innervated muscles and electrodiagnosis for the focal radial nerve injury

Location	Muscles innervated by radial nerve from proximal to distal upper extremity	Nerve	Muscles showing neurogenic change in the crutch palsy (posterior cord injury)	Muscles showing neurogenic change in the Saturday night palsy (spiral groove injury)	Muscles showing neurogenic change in posterior interosseous nerve syndrome
Shoulder	(Deltoid)*	(Axillary)*			
	Triceps	Radial	✓		
Arm	Anconeus	Radial	✓	✓	
Forearm	Brachioradialis	Radial	✓	✓	
	Extensor carpi radialis	Radial	✓	✓	
	Supinator	PIN†	✓	✓	✓
	Extensor carpi ulnaris	PIN†	✓	✓	✓
	Extensor digitorum communis	PIN†	✓	✓	✓
	Extensor digiti minimi	PIN†	✓	✓	✓
	Abductor pollicis longus	PIN†	✓	✓	✓
	Extensor pollicis longus	PIN†	✓	✓	✓
	Extensor pollicis brevis	PIN†	✓	✓	✓
	Extensor indicis	PIN†	✓	✓	✓
Clinical signs	Decreased distal radial sensation		Yes	Yes	No
	Weakness of abduction of shoulder		Yes	No	No
	Weakness of extension of shoulder		Yes	No	No
	Weakness of extension of elbow		Yes	Yes	No
	Weakness of extension of wrist		Yes	Yes	Depends on the location of lesion
	Weakness of extension of MCP		Yes	Yes	Yes
	Weakness of DIP/PIP extension		Yes	Yes	Yes
	Weakness of supination of forearm		Yes	Yes	Depends on the location of lesion

*Deltoid while not radially innervated, is innervated by the axillary nerve, which arises from the posterior cord with the radial nerve.
†Posterior interosseous nerve is a motor branch of radial nerve.

Motor Nerve Conduction Studies

Radial motor studies can be very helpful in diagnosing radial nerve injuries. In axonal injuries, there is a reduction in the compound muscle action potential (CMAP) amplitude after 4–7 days. This can be compared to the contralateral (unaffected) side. Radial conduction velocities may appear to be abnormally fast (e.g., more than 75 meters/second), but the value of doing this study is to look for a *focal conduction block* or decreased *amplitude*. In primarily demyelinating lesions at the spiral groove, the CMAPs recorded at the elbow, forearm and below can be normal. However, stimulation proximal to the spiral groove may reveal marked temporal dispersion or a decrease of amplitude or area (evidence of conduction block).

Late Responses

Late responses are non-specific and not typically done in suspected radial neuropathy.

EMG

The EMG will typically be abnormal in motor axonal radial nerve lesions. It may demonstrate the usual findings in any neuropathy (spontaneous activity, large motor unit action potentials (MUAPs) with long duration, possibly polyphasic in chronic cases, etc.). Since the extensor indicis muscle is the most distal muscle innervated by the radial nerve, it is often tested first. The crux of the EMG study in a radial neuropathy is to locate the lesion by knowing the anatomy.

Table 11.1 is a summary of NCS/EMG findings in radial neuropathy. A muscle innervated by C7, but not by the radial nerve (such as the pronator teres or flexor carpi radialis muscle), should be tested. Such muscles would be normal in a radial nerve injury, but may be abnormal in a C7 radiculopathy. If the radial nerve injury is in the axilla, the triceps muscle may be abnormal, but the deltoid muscle (innervated by the axillary nerve) should be normal. It should also be noted that in patients with a supinator syndrome, the supinator muscle itself would be normal. This is because the radial nerve innervation to the supinator muscle occurs proximally. The radial nerve is compressed in the supinator muscle *after* the supinator has received its innervation.

 ## Summary

In summary, electrodiagnostic findings in radial neuropathy may include (depending on the location of the lesion):

1. decreased amplitude of the radial SNAP
2. decreased amplitude of radial CMAP
3. slowing of radial motor conduction velocity across the affected segment
4. a drop in radial CMAP amplitude across the affected segment (conduction block)
5. spontaneous potentials (fibs and PSWs in radially innervated muscles distal to lesion)
6. if the posterior interosseous nerve (a motor branch) is affected, the radial CMAP may be abnormal, but the radial SNAP should be normal (this may be seen in the supinator syndrome).
7. if the superficial radial sensory nerve (a pure sensory nerve) is affected, the radial SNAP may be abnormal, but the radial CMAP should be normal.

12

Radiculopathy

Lyn Weiss, Nancy Fung

Radiculopathy is a lesion of a specific nerve root and is generally caused by root compression. It is second only to carpal tunnel syndrome (CTS), as the reason for referral for electrodiagnostic study. The diagnosis of radiculopathy is based on a patient's history, physical examination, and electrodiagnostic study. Imaging studies are also helpful. The diagnosis of radiculopathy is contingent upon motor and sensory symptoms and/or findings in a distribution consistent with a nerve root. In certain clear-cut clinical pictures, electrodiagnosis may not be necessary.

Often however, in the case of a radiculopathy or possible radiculopathy, electrodiagnostic studies are quite helpful in making or confirming the diagnosis, as well as in determining the prognosis. Whereas an MRI may be helpful in anatomically localizing a lesion it is basically only a snapshot in time. On the other hand, although an EMG does not reveal the anatomy in the same way that imaging studies do, it provides physiological information about what is actually occurring to the nerves and muscles. Therefore, *both* imaging studies (usually an MRI) and electrodiagnostic studies are extremely helpful in confirming the diagnosis of a radiculopathy.

 ## Clinical Presentation

Patients with radiculopathy will frequently complain of neck pain radiating to the arm (cervical radiculopathy) or back pain radiating to the leg (lumbosacral radiculopathy). There may also be numbness or tingling in the distribution of a sensory nerve root, referred to as a *dermatomal* distribution (see Fig. 18.2). Thoracic radiculopathies, while rare, would radiate pain and/or numbness in the distribution of the nerve root. In addition, if the motor fibers are affected, there will be weakness of muscles innervated by that nerve root, referred to as a *myotomal* distribution (Tables 12.2 and 12.3). For example, a patient with a right L5 radiculopathy may complain of back pain radiating to the right leg, numbness along the lateral aspect of the right leg into the dorsum of the foot, and foot slap with walking.

On physical examination, the patient described above may have normal reflexes, decreased sensation on the lateral aspect of the right leg and dorsum of the right foot, and weakness of the ankle dorsiflexors. It is important to remember that not all patients experience the same symptoms. In addition, dermatomal and myotomal distributions may vary amongst individuals. It is possible for a radiculopathy to affect predominantly sensory fibers, motor fibers, or both. Physical findings that may suggest a radiculopathy include the following:

- decreased reflexes in muscles innervated by that nerve root
- weakness in muscles innervated by that nerve root
- sensory symptoms in a dermatomal distribution.

Table 12.1 Levels of confidence in diagnosis of cervical or lumbosacral radiculopathy

EMG diagnosis:	Mildly suggestive	Moderately suggestive	Strongly suggestive/ definitive
Muscles with neurogenic change	Early change in paraspinals or one root innervated muscle without motor/sensory NCS change	Early change in . paraspinals and two or more same root innervated muscles without motor/sensory NCS change. Acute denervation and/or chronic change on paraspinals and any one spinal root innervated muscle	Acute denervation and/or chronic change in two muscles from two different peripheral nerves but same myotome as well as paraspinal involvement

The physical examination has several limitations that may make electromyography a necessary adjunct in the diagnosis of radiculopathy. A mild weakness can be easily missed on manual muscle testing. If the patient is stronger than the examiner, subtle weakness in the upper extremities may not be apparent. The examination is not quantitative and a loss of 10 pounds of biceps strength, for example, may be imperceptible. Lower extremity muscles such as the quadriceps can exert forces greater than the total body weight and only severe weakness will be apparent. In many cases of clinically missed weakness, electromyography will be positive. For instance a 10% loss of motor axons may reveal no perceptible weakness on physical examination. However, EMG testing is likely to be sensitive enough to detect the abnormality.

 Anatomy

Electrodiagnostic evaluation of a radiculopathy requires a thorough knowledge of the anatomy of the spine. There are 31 pairs of spinal nerves attached to the spinal cord by ventral and dorsal roots. The spinal nerve is a mixed sensory and motor nerve that is formed by the fusion of ventral and dorsal roots in the intervertebral foramina (see Fig. 1.1).

- The *ventral* roots are axons with cell bodies in the anterior horn cells in the ventral gray matter of the spinal cord. These roots are from motor neurons whose axons terminate in a neuromuscular junction.
- The *dorsal* roots are axons with cell bodies in the dorsal root ganglia in the vertebral foramina, outside the spinal cord. These are sensory axons.

The cell body of sensory fibers is outside the spinal cord, as opposed to motor fibers where the cell body is within the spinal cord. In a radiculopathy there is usually continuity between the sensory cell body and the digits, as the lesion is proximal to the dorsal root ganglia. Although sensation may be altered, electrodiagnostically the sensory nerve action potential (SNAP) will not be affected (see Fig. 1.1).

All the muscles that are innervated by a single ventral root define a myotome. A dermatome is the sensory distribution of a single nerve root. Except for the rhomboid muscle, which is predominantly innervated by the C5 root, almost every muscle is innervated by multiple roots and is therefore part of multiple myotomes. It should be

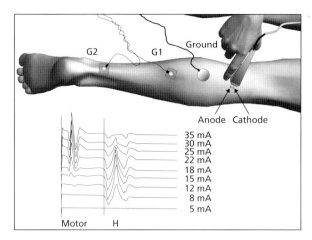

Figure 12.1
Assessment for S1 radiculopathy by performing an H-reflex.

kept in mind when performing a physical examination that dermatomes (the skin area innervated by a single dorsal root) also overlap.

 ## Electrodiagnostic Medicine Evaluation

Sensory Nerve Conduction Studies

Pain, numbness, and tingling are common complaints in patients with radiculopathy. However, in the majority of radicular processes, the SNAP should be normal, both in amplitude and latency. Latency is contingent on the speed of the fastest fibers. Amplitude is contingent on the number of fibers firing. Damage to the myelin sheath of an axon would generally cause slowing or conduction block. This would be apparent on nerve studies if the lesion were between the area of stimulation and the pickup electrodes.

In radiculopathy, any demyelination is proximal to the area being stimulated and therefore conduction block or slowing will not be seen. Basically this means that *sensory NCS are always normal unless there is alternate or coexisting pathology*, e.g., carpal tunnel syndrome. When there is axonal damage and the distal parts of the axon are no longer contiguous with the cell body, the axon will die back, a process known as Wallerian degeneration. In a radiculopathy any damage to the dorsal (sensory) fibers is generally proximal to the dorsal root ganglion. Therefore as the axon is still in contact with its cell body, no sensory denervation will occur. Even in severe lesions that would result in anesthesia, normal sensory studies can be seen. If SNAP abnormalities are found, it is important to rule out other lesions such as a brachial plexopathy, an entrapment neuropathy or a peripheral neuropathy.

Motor Nerve Conduction Studies

Compound muscle action potential (CMAP) amplitudes reflect the actual number of motor fibers activated upon stimulation. The latency is a function of the speed of the fastest fibers. *In general, both the sensory and motor NCS will be normal in an isolated case of radiculopathy*. However, in a severe radicular lesion (which is distal to the anterior horn cell) axonal loss can result in Wallerian degeneration distal to the lesion. Therefore the

CMAP amplitude might be reduced. On the other hand, if it is a focal demyelinating lesion, the amplitude will be normal.

Nonetheless even with a lesion that causes axonal degeneration, the CMAP amplitude could still be normal. This is because the muscles have input from multiple nerve roots and motor units. The radicular lesion may impinge on nerve fibers that do not innervate the muscle being tested, or fibers from other nerve roots may contribute more significantly and therefore the amplitude will not be significantly affected. For example, if the C8 nerve root is affected, the amplitude of a CMAP recorded from the abductor pollicis brevis (APB) muscle is usually not affected. In addition to receiving fibers from C8, the APB receives innervation from T1 and is probably more heavily innnervated by T1 than C8. Since the lesion is proximal to the area being stimulated, no slowing or conduction block should be present on motor nerve studies.

From these discussions, it should be apparent that motor and sensory studies are of limited use in radiculopathies. When abnormalities occur they are likely to be of motor nerve (CMAP) amplitude. Increased distal latencies and slowing or conduction block or decreased SNAP amplitude would not suggest radiculopathy but would suggest an alternate diagnosis. In fact, the main value of nerve conduction studies in testing for radiculopathy is to *rule out* other diagnoses such as a peripheral or entrapment neuropathy.

Late Responses

The *H-reflex* is a monosynaptic or oligosynaptic spinal reflex involving both motor and sensory fibers. It electrically tests some of the same fibers as are tested in the ankle jerk reflexes. In fact it is rare to be unable to obtain an H-reflex in the presence of an ankle jerk reflex. If this occurs, technical factors should be considered. In theory it is a sensitive measure in assessing radiculopathy because: it helps to assess proximal lesions, it becomes abnormal relatively early in the development of radiculopathy, and it incorporates sensory fiber function proximal to the dorsal root ganglion. *The H-reflex primarily assesses afferent and efferent S1 fibers.* Clinically, L5 and S1 radiculopathies may appear similar on EMG due to the overlap of myotomes. The H-reflex's primary value is in distinguishing S1 from L5 radiculopathies.

When assessing for S1 radiculopathy, the H-reflex latency is recorded from the gastrocnemius-soleus muscle group upon stimulating the tibial nerve in the popliteal fossa (Fig. 12.1). The H-reflex is elicited with a submaximal stimulation with the cathode proximal to the anode. As the stimulation is gradually increased from peak H-amplitude, we generally see a diminishment of the H-amplitude with a concurrent increase in the M-wave amplitude. With supramaximal stimulation, the H-reflex is usually absent.

The H-reflex can also be used in C6/C7 radiculopathy by recording over the flexor carpi radialis muscle and stimulating the median nerve at the elbow. The median H-reflex is less commonly performed and clinically is less likely to be helpful for radiculopathy than a lower extremity H-reflex. *Generally, gastrocnemius-soleus H-reflex latency side-to-side differences of greater than 1.5 ms are suggestive of S1 radiculopathy.*

Although the H-reflex is sensitive, it has certain limitations. First, patients with an S1 radiculopathy can have a normal H-reflex. Second, an abnormal H-reflex is only suggestive, but not definitive for radiculopathy because the abnormality may originate in other components of the long pathway involved, such as the peripheral nerves, plexuses, or spinal cord. Third, once the H-reflex becomes abnormal, it usually does not return to normal, even over time. Finally, the H-reflex is often absent in otherwise normal individuals over the age of 60 years. The reflexes therefore can be considered a sensitive, but not specific indicator of pathology. Latency of the H-reflex is dependent on the age and leg length of the patient (see Table 4.1). A side-to-side amplitude difference of 60% or more may also indicate pathology.

F-waves are low amplitude late responses thought to be due to antidromic activation of motor neurons (anterior horn cells) following peripheral nerve stimulation, which then cause orthodromic impulses to pass back along the involved motor axons. Some electromyographers have called this a 'backfiring' of axons. It is called the F-wave because it was first noted in intrinsic foot muscles. The F-wave has small amplitude, a variable configuration, and a variable latency. Generally F-wave amplitudes are on the order of 1% of the orthodromically generated motor response (M-response). The most widely used parameter is the latency of the shortest reproducible response. The F-wave can be found in many muscles of the upper and lower extremities. Unfortunately F-waves have not turned out to be as sensitive a test as initially hoped. The reasons for this are:

1. the pathways involve only the motor fibers
2. as with the H-reflex, it involves a long neuronal pathway so that if there is a focal lesion it might be obscured
3. if an abnormality is present, the F-wave will not pinpoint the exact cause because any lesion, from the anterior horn cell to the muscle being tested, can affect the F-wave similarly
4. since muscles have multiple root innervations, the shortest latency may reflect the healthy fibers in the non-affected root and
5. the latency and amplitude of an F-wave is variable so that multiple stimulations must be performed to find the shortest latency.

If not enough stimulations are done (usually more than 10), the shortest latency may not be apparent. Thus, use of F-waves in evaluating for radiculopathy are extremely limited and should not be the basis upon which a diagnosis is made. See Table 4.2 for a comparison of H-reflex and F-waves.

EMG

EMG still is the most useful procedure in localizing radiculopathy and predicting prognosis. In cases of radiculopathy causing axonal damage, Wallerian degeneration will occur. Muscle fibers supplied by these axons will begin to fire spontaneously. This spontaneous activity in the form of fibrillation potentials and positive sharp waves initially occurs proximally, and extends distally with time. These potentials have a characteristic appearance and sound.

The presence of spontaneous activity is the most objective evidence of acute denervation. Lesser lesions can cause increased insertional activity although the subjective nature in determining these lowers the confidence level in diagnosis. In reinnervation and with sprouting of collateral axons, motor unit abnormalities such as long duration polyphasic motor units may be present. The diagnosis of radiculopathy should not be made based solely on polyphasicity. Much of the work on polyphasicity was based on studies with concentric electrodes that record from a smaller area than monopolar electrodes and are less likely to see polyphasic potentials.

Recruitment abnormalities, if seen, would be typical of a neuropathic recruitment including few motor units firing at a high rate (higher than 20 Hz) as described in Chapter 5.

Spontaneous activity as seen by EMG begins in the proximal paraspinal muscles, within 5–7 days of compression. Most limb muscles show spontaneous activity within

3 weeks, but 5–6 weeks may be required in the distal portions of the limb.[1] Similarly, reinnervation occurs proximally first, with paraspinal muscle reinnervation thought to occur after 6–9 weeks, followed by the proximal muscles at 2–5 months, and the distal muscles at 3–7 months.[2] One should keep in mind that EMG in general will be able to assess only axonal injury to motor fibers.

The selection of muscles to be tested is of critical importance. The needle examination should be sufficiently detailed to distinguish between lesions at the root, plexus, and peripheral nerve level. The muscles noted to be weak on examination, or muscles with abnormal reflexes, should be examined in order to maximize the yield of the study. In fact, the physical examination serves as the foundation upon which the electrodiagnostic study is performed. Without an adequate history and physical exam, the yield of the electrodiagnostic studies is significantly lowered. There is not enough time and it would be unkind to your patient to attempt to examine every possible muscle. Therefore the study needs to be tailored to fit the specific clinical circumstances.

Table 12.2 Clinical picture – cervical radiculopathy[3,4]

Root level	Muscle group	Clinical sign
C5	Rhomboid (dorsal scapular nerve) Supraspinatus/infraspinatus (suprascapular nerve) Deltoid/teres minor (axillary nerve) Biceps brachii/brachialis (musculocutaneous nerve)	1. Positive neck distraction/compression test 2. Decreased/absent biceps tendon reflex 3. Decreased/absent sensation to the lateral arm (axillary nerve) 4. Weakness of shoulder abduction
C6	Extensor carpi radialis longus and brevis (radial nerve) Pronator teres/flexor carpi radialis (median nerve) Deltoid/teres minor (axillary nerve)	1. Decreased/absent brachioradialis reflex 2. Decreased/absent sensation to the lateral forearm (musculocutaneous nerve) 3. Weakness of wrist extension
C7	Triceps/extensor digitorum communis/extensor indicis proprius digiti minimi (radial nerve) Flexor carpi radialis (median nerve) Flexor carpi ulnaris (ulnar nerve)	1. Decreased/absent triceps reflex 2. Decreased/absent sensation to the middle finger 3. Weakness of wrist flexion
C8	Flexor carpi ulnaris (ulnar nerve) Flexor pollicis longus/flexor digitorum superficialis (median nerve) Flexor digitorum profundus (median or ulnar nerve) Extensor indicis proprius/extensor pollicis brevis (radial nerve) First dorsal interosseous (ulnar nerve)	1. Decreased/absent sensation to the ring and little fingers of the hand and to the distal half of the forearm's ulnar side (ulnar nerve) 2. Weakness of finger flexion 3. Intrinsic weakness and atrophy
T1	Abductor pollicis brevis (median nerve) Abductor digiti minimi/dorsal interosseous (ulnar nerve)	1. Decreased/absent sensation to medial side of the upper half of the forearm and the arm (medial brachial cutaneous nerve) 2. Weakness of finger abduction/adduction

In order to have a definitive diagnosis of radiculopathy, a *paraspinal muscle and two muscles from different peripheral nerves innervated by the same root should have positive findings*. If only some (but not all) of the criteria are met, the diagnosis of radiculopathy is only suggestive (see Table 12.2). It is also important to note that *if the patient only has sensory involvement, the NCS/EMG test may be completely normal*. Remember that the SNAP will not be affected, and the EMG only assesses motor fibers. In these cases the EMG may be performed to rule out other causes for the patient's symptoms. The report should specify that while the study is normal, radiculopathy cannot be ruled out, and it may be appropriate to refer for other diagnostic tests.

Table 12.3 Clinical picture – lumbosacral radiculopathy[3,4]

Root level	Muscles	Clinical sign
L2, 3,4*	Iliacus/vastus medialis (femoral nerve) L2, 3 Adductor longus/gracilis (obturator nerve) L2, 3,4	Pain in the thigh Weakness in hip flexion, adduction
(L4)	Vastus lateralis, rectus femorus Tibialis anterior (deep peroneal nerve) L4–L5 Vastus medialis and lateralis (L2–4)	Decreased/absent patellar reflex** Pain in the medial side of the leg Knee extension weakness
L5	Gluteus medius/tensor fasciae latae (superior gluteal nerve L4–S2, posterior) Flexor hallucis longus/flexor digitorum longus/lateral gastrocnemius/tibialis posterior (tibial nerve, L5–S2)/tibialis anterior Extensor hallucis longus/extensor digitorum longus (deep peroneal nerve, L5)	Pain & paresthesias in lateral aspect of leg and dorsum of foot Ankle dorsiflexor weakness
S1***	Medial gastrocnemius/soleus/ flexor hallucis brevis (tibial nerve, L5–S2) Peroneus longus and brevis (superficial peroneal nerve, L5, S1)/tensor fascia lata/gluteus maximus (superior/inferior gluteal nerve L4–S1/ L5–S2) Extensor hallucis longus, extensor digitorum (deep peroneal nerve, L4, L5, S1)	Decreased/absent ankle reflex Pain & paresthesias to the lateral border of the foot Weakness of foot plantar flexion and toe extension

*Lesions of L2, L3, and L4 are best considered collectively because they have such extensive myotomal overlap. Consequently, it is frequently impossible to distinguish isolated lesions involving one of them. It can be difficult to diagnose an L2 or an L3 radiculopathy: The L2–L3 myotomes have limited limb representation. All the muscles innervated by the L2–L3 myotomes are located proximally in the lower extremity and they are reinnervated sooner than muscles located more distally. There is no reliable sensory NCS available for evaluating the L2–L4 fibers. In L4 radiculopathies similar changes may be found in the tibialis anterior muscle, but their absence never excludes a lesion of that root.
**The patellar reflex is a deep tendon reflex, mediated through nerves emanating from the L2, L3, and L4 nerve roots, but predominantly from L4. For clinical application, the patellar reflex is considered an L4 reflex; however, even if the L4 nerve root is totally cut, the reflex can still be present in significantly diminished form.
***H-reflex may confirm diagnosis and distinguish S1 from L5 radiculopathy.

Summary

In summary, electrodiagnostic findings in radiculopathy may include:

1. normal SNAP amplitudes
2. normal CMAP (predominantly)
3. spontaneous potentials (fibs and PSWs) in the paraspinal muscles and two muscles from different peripheral nerves innervated by the same affected root level.

See Tables 12.2 and 12.3 for a summary of clinical findings in radiculopathy.

REFERENCES

1. Dumitru D, Zwarts MJ. Radiculopathies. In Dumitru D, Amato AA, Zwarts M, eds. Electrodiagnostic Medicine, 2nd Edn. Philadelphia: Hanley & Belfus, 2002, pp. 713–776.
2. Johnson EW. Electrodiagnosis of Radiculopathy. In Johnson EW, ed. Practical Electromyography, 2nd Edn. Baltimore: Williams and Wilkins, 1988, pp. 229–245.
3. Wilbourn AJ. AAEM mimimonograph #32: The electrodiagnostic examination in patients with radiculopathies. Muscle & Nerve 1998; 21: 1612–1631.
4. Dumitru D. In Dumitru D, Amato AA, Zwarts M, eds. Electrodiagnostic Medicine, 2nd Edn. Philadelphia: Hanley & Belfus, 2002, pp. 523–584.

13

Spinal Stenosis

Lyn Weiss

 Clinical presentation

Spinal stenosis can be defined as narrowing or restriction of the vertebral canal, and can affect any spinal level. The spinal cord, cauda equina, and/or nerve root structures may be involved.

Patients with spinal stenosis usually complain of back or neck pain with radiation to one or both extremities. Patients with lumbar stenosis usually complain of a dull ache in the hip and thigh region. The pain is typically relieved with sitting, which tends to flex the spine and therefore increases the diameter of the spinal canal. This is referred to as *neurogenic claudication*. (In true vascular claudication, the patient only has to stop and rest to relieve the symptoms, not necessarily sit down.)

 Anatomy

The lumbar spinal canal usually has an anteroposterior diameter of about 15 mm or more. Any decrease in the diameter of the canal beyond 12 mm is considered significant for spinal stenosis. The condition may be due to congenital or acquired factors. These factors can include spondylolisthesis, enlargement of the soft tissues in and around the canal, hypertrophy of the facet joints, intervertebral disc herniation, or ligamentum flavum hypertrophy or laxity.

 Electrodiagnostic findings

Although electrodiagnostic testing in spinal stenosis may be non-specific, testing is helpful to rule out other causes for the patient's symptoms, including radiculopathy, peripheral neuropathy or entrapment neuropathy. It is important to note that electro-diagnostic studies are not typically done as a means of diagnosing spinal stenosis. This diagnosis is usually made with information from the history, physical examination and imaging studies.

Sensory Nerve Conduction Studies

Sensory nerve conduction studies and amplitudes should be *normal* in spinal stenosis. This is due to the fact that the sensory (dorsal) root ganglion is located outside the spinal canal and therefore usually not affected in spinal stenosis. In summary, similar to radiculopathies, sensory and motor NCS are typically normal with the exception of severe axonal loss, in which case you may see decreased amplitude of the CMAP.

Motor Nerve Conduction Studies

Motor nerve studies should demonstrate normal distal latencies, as the distal aspect of the nerve is not affected. Velocities and amplitudes are usually unaffected, unless the disease has progressed to the point that there is significant axonal damage and motor axon collateral sprouting cannot keep pace with axonal damage. In such cases, you may see decreased amplitude of the CMAP on nerve conduction studies.

Late Responses

H-reflexes may be prolonged or absent bilaterally if the S1 nerve root is affected by the spinal stenosis. F-waves are generally not helpful in the evaluation of spinal stenosis as they are non-specific.

EMG

If neural compression is significant, you may see multilevel bilateral abnormalities, including fibrillations and positive sharp waves (in acute neural compression), and large amplitude, polyphasic, increased duration motor unit action potentials (in chronic neural compression). It is important to test multiple bilateral paraspinal levels as well as multiple myotomal levels in both extremities.

Summary

The classic electrodiagnostic findings in spinal stenosis may include:

1. Normal SNAP amplitudes and conduction velocities
2. Normal CMAP latency, amplitude and conduction velocities
3. EMG findings of bilateral multilevel nerve root involvement.

14

Peroneal Neuropathy

Julie Silver

 ## Clinical Presentation

Peroneal neuropathy is the most common mononeuropathy in the legs and occurs due to compression, entrapment, ischemia or direct trauma. The most likely site of compression is at the fibular neck (or head), where the nerve is very superficial (Fig. 14.1). The patient typically presents with foot drop that is usually acute but may be gradual. There may be a history of recent falls or trips as well. Paresthesias and numbness in the lower lateral leg and dorsum of the foot may be present. Pain is typically absent.

A thorough history can help determine the cause of the symptoms (e.g., a plaster cast that was too tight, a habit of crossing the legs, a brace that doesn't fit well, occupational squatting such as in a carpenter, etc.). Peroneal neuropathy can easily be confused with lumbar radiculopathy (usually L5), sciatic neuropathy or lumbosacral plexopathy. Electrodiagnostic studies can be crucial to determining the location and extent of damage.

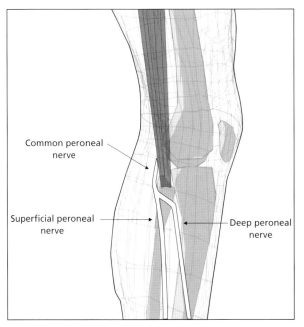

Figure 14.1
Peroneal nerve.

Common peroneal nerve

Superficial peroneal nerve

Deep peroneal nerve

In peroneal neuropathy, both the deep and superficial peroneal nerves are usually affected. In cases where only one branch is affected, deep peroneal neuropathy is more common than superficial peroneal neuropathy. The physical examination will vary depending on the affected nerve(s) (Fig. 14.2). Since the deep peroneal nerve provides sensation to the first dorsal web space, assessment of sensory deficits in this region can help localize the lesion. Strength deficits are usually most notable in ankle dorsiflexion and great toe extension. There may be a foot slap or steppage gait when the patient ambulates. Reflexes are typically normal. Tinel's sign may be present over the fibular neck.

Anatomy

The common peroneal nerve arises from the L4–S1 nerve roots that travel through the lumbosacral plexus and then through the sciatic nerve. Within the sciatic nerve, the fibers that eventually form the common peroneal nerve run separately from those that distally become the tibial nerve (separation of these nerves usually occurs at the level of the popliteal fossa). The common peroneal nerve branches, giving rise to the lateral cutaneous nerve of the knee and then winds around the fibular neck and passes through the 'fibular tunnel' between the peroneus longus muscle and the fibula. It then divides into superficial and deep branches. The superficial peroneal nerve innervates the peroneus longus and brevis and terminates in sensory branches that supply the lateral aspect of the lower leg and the dorsum of the foot and toes. In 15–25% of people, the superficial peroneal nerve also gives rise to the *accessory peroneal nerve*. This provides an anomalous innervation of the extensor digitorum brevis (see Chapter 8, Pitfalls).

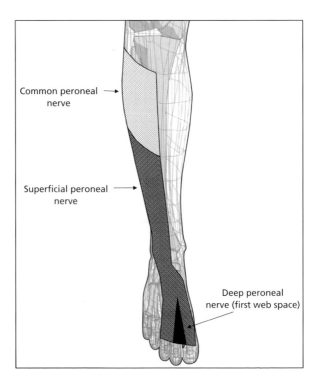

Figure 14.2
Sensory distribution of peroneal nerve.

Common peroneal nerve →

Superficial peroneal nerve →

Deep peroneal nerve (first web space)

The deep peroneal nerve (also called the anterior tibial nerve) supplies the tibialis anterior, extensor digitorum longus, extensor hallucis longus, peroneus tertius and extensor digitorum brevis. The terminal sensory branches supply the skin over the first web space.

The peroneal division of the sciatic nerve innervates the short head of the biceps femoris. This is important electrodiagnostically as it is the only muscle proximal to the knee that is innervated by the peroneal nerve. In peroneal neuropathy at the fibular neck, the short head of the biceps femoris muscle should not be affected.

 ## Electrodiagnostic Findings

Sensory Nerve Conduction Studies

The superficial sensory peroneal nerve study is not significantly more technically demanding than the sural sensory study; however, it is often not done. Nevertheless, when there is a question of a peroneal neuropathy, it is an important study to perform. In lesions that are axonal or mixed axonal and demyelinating, the superficial peroneal SNAP amplitude is low or absent. However, in purely demyelinating lesions at the fibular neck, the distal superficial peroneal sensory response remains normal.

Motor Nerve Conduction Studies

In demyelinating lesions, focal slowing or conduction block can be noted in peroneal motor studies across the fibular neck. Proximal slowing of more than 10 meters per second compared to the distal conduction velocity is considered significant. A drop in amplitude of the peroneal CMAP of more than 20% suggests conduction block.

If axonal loss is predominantly present, then peroneal CMAP amplitudes will be reduced at all stimulation sites (e.g., ankle, below the fibular head and lateral popliteal fossa). The motor nerve conduction velocity and the distal latency may be slightly slowed or normal – depending on whether the fastest conducting axons have been lost. Often there is a combination of demyelination and axonal loss in the same patient.

The extensor digitorum brevis (EDB) is usually the site of recording for motor studies. However, it is not unusual for the EDB to be atrophied for non-pathologic reasons (e.g., due to wearing tight shoes). Therefore, although the EDB is the usual site of recording, it may be worthwhile to consider recording over the tibialis anterior muscle (TA). If you do the study over the EDB and it does not show focal slowing or conduction block, then consider repeating the study using the active electrode over the tibialis anterior, which may pick up the deficit. Of course, if there is any question of an abnormal study, you can compare it to the contralateral side as well.

Late Responses

In peroneal neuropathy at the fibular neck, F-wave responses may be prolonged or absent on the affected side and normal on the unaffected side. However, these responses are non-specific and should not be used to diagnose peroneal neuropathy. H-reflexes are usually done to rule out an alternate diagnosis and should be normal in peroneal neuropathy.

EMG

EMG is abnormal in axonal peroneal lesions when a significant axonotmesis is present. Abnormalities will be found in peroneal-innervated muscles. In axonal lesions, there will be evidence of spontaneous activity, positive sharp waves and fibrillation potentials,

Table 14.1 Muscle involvement in focal peroneal nerve injury

Location	Muscles innervated by peroneal nerve from proximal to distal lower extremity	Nerve	Neurogenic change in muscles in peroneal nerve injury above fibular head/sciatic nerve injury in buttock	Neurogenic change in muscles in peroneal nerve injury to the fibular head	Neurogenic change in muscles in deep peroneal neuropathy	Neurogenic change in muscles in the superficial peroneal neuropathy
Thigh	Biceps femoris (short head)	SN-P*	✓			
Leg	Extensor digitorum longus	DP*	✓	✓	✓	
	Tibialis anterior	DP*	✓	✓	✓	
	Extensor hallucis longus	DP*	✓	✓	✓	
	Peroneus tertius	DP*	✓	✓	✓	
	Extensor digitorum brevis	DP*	✓	✓	✓	
	Peroneus longus	SP*	✓	✓		✓
	Peroneus brevis	SP*	✓	✓		✓
Clinical sign:	Foot drop, weakness of foot dorsiflexion, high-stepping gait		Yes	Yes	Yes	No
	Weakness of foot eversion		Yes	Yes	No	Yes
	Pain, loss of sensation or numbness		Anterolateral part of the leg up to lateral side of the popliteal fossa and/or the dorsum of the foot**	Anterolateral part of the leg and the dorsum of the foot†	A small area between the first and second toes‡	Most of the foot's dorsum except the region between the first and second toes
	Tinel's sign may be present		No	Fib head	No	No

*DP – deep peroneal nerve; SP – superficial peroneal nerve; SN-P sciatic nerve, peroneal division.

**Lateral cutaneous nerve of the calf.

†Lateral and medial terminal branches of superficial peroneal nerve.

‡Terminal branches of DPN.

See:
Leis AA. Atlas of Electromyography. Oxford: Oxford University Press, 2000, pp. 135–145.
Dumitru D, Amato AA, Zwarts M, eds. Electrodiagnostic Medicine, 2nd Edn. Philadelphia: Hanley & Belfus, 2002, pp. 898–905.

and decreased recruitment of motor unit action potentials (MUAPs). In chronic axonal lesions there may be evidence of decreased recruitment of MUAPs and the morphology of the MUAPs may be long duration, high-amplitude and polyphasic. In predominantly demyelinating lesions, only decreased MUAP recruitment will occur and the MUAP morphology will be normal. The EMG is important in order to rule out other nerve lesions. Therefore, proximal leg and paraspinal muscles are often tested (to rule out a radiculopathy) and tibial-innervated muscles are sampled below the knee. It is important to note that the tibial nerve supplies the hamstring muscles, with the exception of the peroneal innervated short head of the biceps femoris muscle.

The short head of the biceps femoris can be very helpful in distinguishing a peroneal nerve injury at the fibular head from a sciatic nerve injury affecting predominantly peroneal fibers. Due to the anatomy of the sciatic nerve (as noted above) the peroneal fibers can be more susceptible to injury than the tibial (especially in the sciatic notch and buttock region). In instances where insults could have occurred to the buttock region as well as the fibular head (i.e., trauma, foot drop after hip surgery) the short head of the biceps femoris may be the main distinguishing factor between these lesions.

 ## Summary

The classic electrodiagnostic findings in a peroneal neuropathy at the fibular neck may include:

1. Reduced peroneal CMAP amplitude compared to the contralateral side
2. Peroneal motor nerve conduction block or focal slowing across the fibular neck
3. Reduced superficial peroneal SNAP amplitude
4. Absent or prolonged peroneal F-response on the affected side
5. Normal sural sensory, tibial motor and H-reflexes
6. EMG findings of spontaneous activity and/or reinnervation in muscles supplied by the deep and superficial peroneal nerves
7. Normal EMG findings in the short head of the biceps femoris, paraspinal muscles and tibially innervated muscles.

See Table 14.1 for a summary of electrodiagnostic findings in peroneal neuropathy.

15

Tarsal Tunnel Syndrome

Julie Silver

Clinical Presentation

Tarsal tunnel syndrome is an entrapment neuropathy of the tibial nerve behind the medial malleolus. The syndrome is much less common than other neuropathies such as carpal tunnel syndrome or peroneal neuropathy. This neuropathy is nearly always unilateral. Conditions that may lead to tarsal tunnel syndrome include trauma, space-occupying lesions, biomechanical problems causing joint deformity and systemic diseases. Some cases are idiopathic as well.

Patients with tarsal tunnel syndrome generally complain of pain around the ankle (especially medially) and/or paresthesias typically accompanied by numbness over the sole of the foot. Weakness in the foot is not very common in this neuropathy.

On physical examination there may be a positive Tinel's sign over the tibial nerve at the medial ankle (Fig. 15.1). Sensory exam might be abnormal over the plantar surface of the foot. Subtle weakness is not well appreciated because it is often difficult to isolate the muscles supplied by the involved nerve(s).

Anatomy

Tarsal tunnel syndrome involves entrapment of the *tibial nerve* or any of its branches in the region beneath the flexor retinaculum at the medial ankle. In addition to the tibial nerve, the tibial artery and tendons of the flexor hallucis longus, flexor digitorum longus

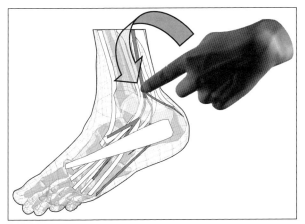

Figure 15.1
Tinel's sign over the tibial nerve.

and tibialis posterior muscles pass through the tarsal tunnel (see Fig. 15.2). The tibial nerve divides into two sensory branches (medial and lateral calcaneal sensory nerves) and two mixed motor and sensory branches (medial and lateral plantar nerves). These nerves supply the medial and lateral sole of the foot respectively.

Both plantar nerves innervate the intrinsic muscles of the foot. The medial plantar nerve typically supplies the first three toes and the medial half of the fourth toe, while the lateral plantar nerve supplies the lateral fourth toe and the entire fifth toe.

 ## Electrodiagnostic Findings

Sensory Nerve Conduction Studies

In tarsal tunnel syndrome, the medial and lateral plantar sensory nerve action potential (SNAP) may be affected or absent. However, this should be interpreted with caution since pure SNAPs are difficult to obtain in the foot and frequently require averaging. Also, the foot is very sensitive to temperature changes. It is important to note that medial and lateral plantar sensory nerves are often hard to obtain even in normal patients.

Mixed and Motor Nerve Conduction Studies

These are the most common and important studies done in tarsal tunnel syndrome. The distal latency of the medial plantar nerve or the lateral plantar nerve, or both, may be increased in tarsal tunnel syndrome if demyelination is present. Since motor latencies are less temperature sensitive than sensory latencies, you can compare medial and lateral latencies and compare both latencies to the contralateral (unaffected) side. If axonal loss is prominent, then the compound muscle action potential (CMAP) will be reduced and the distal latencies will be normal or just slightly prolonged.

Late Responses

F-waves may be abnormal but are non-specific and not typically done in tarsal tunnel syndrome studies. H-reflexes should be normal in tarsal tunnel syndrome.

Figure 15.2
Anatomy of the
tibial nerve.

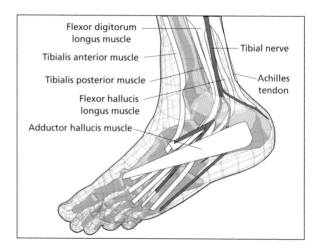

Table 15.1 Muscle involvement in focal tibial nerve injury

Location	Muscles innervated by tibial nerve	Nerve involved	Neurogenic changes in tibial nerve injury above the knee	Neurogenic change on muscles in the tarsal tunnel syndrome*
Leg	Gastrocnemius	Tibial nerve	✓	
	Popliteus	Tibial nerve	✓	
	Soleus	Tibial nerve	✓	
	Tibialis posterior	Tibial nerve	✓	
	Flexor hallucis longus	Tibial nerve	✓	
	Flexor digitorum longus	Tibial nerve	✓	
Foot	Abductor digiti minimi	Lateral plantar nerve	✓	✓
	Quadratus plantae	Lateral plantar nerve	✓	✓
	Flexor digiti min mi	Lateral plantar nerve	✓	✓
	Dorsal interossei	Lateral plantar nerve	✓	✓
	Plantar interossei	Lateral plantar nerve	✓	✓
	Adductor hallucis	Lateral plantar nerve	✓	✓
	Lumbrical	Medial plantar nerve	✓	✓
	Abductor hallucis	Medial plantar nerve	✓	✓
	Flexor digitorum brevis	Medial plantar nerve	✓	
Clinical sign	Nocturnal paresthesias		Variable	Common
	Burning in the sole of the foot		Variable	Common
	Tinel's sign over the tarsal tunnel		No	Common
	Inability of plantar flexion		Variable	No
	Decreased sensation in plantar aspect of the foot		Common	Common

*Tarsal tunnel syndrome is caused by compression of the tibial nerve or its branches at the tarsal tunnel.

EMG

EMG of the foot is usually quite difficult in part because patients tolerate this exam poorly (due to pain). Additionally many patients have difficulty isolating specific muscles for activation. Even in normal people there is often evidence of spontaneous activity as well as long duration and large amplitude MUAPs in foot muscles. Nevertheless, it is recommended that you perform an EMG in tibial innervated muscles both above and below the level of the tarsal tunnel, and that you check peroneal innervated muscles as part of the differential diagnosis. If a positive finding is noted, be sure to check the unaffected foot to rule out the possibility of a normal variant.

 ## Summary

In summary, electrodiagnostic findings in tarsal tunnel syndrome may include:

1. prolonged or low amplitude medial or lateral plantar sensory or mixed nerves responses
2. prolonged distal latency of the medial or lateral plantar motor nerve
3. decreased amplitude of the medial or lateral plantar motor nerve
4. spontaneous potentials (fibs and PSWs) in muscles innervated by lateral or medial plantar nerve.

See Table 15.1 for a summary of NCS/EMG findings in tarsal tunnel syndrome.

16

Peripheral Neuropathy

Lyn Weiss

Peripheral neuropathies occur when there is a *generalized* dysfunction of nerves. This is really a collection of disorders that all have the common characteristic of affecting the peripheral nerves. When doing electrodiagnostic testing on patients with suspected peripheral neuropathy, it is possible to state if a peripheral neuropathy exists, how severe it is, and what the characteristics of the neuropathy are. Based on the characteristics of the neuropathy (axonal, demyelinating, sensory, motor, etc.) the electromyographer can direct the referring clinician towards suspected causes for the neuropathy (Table 16.1).

Clinical Presentation

Symptoms of peripheral neuropathy usually begin in the feet with numbness and/or pain/paresthesias. As the disease progresses, patients may report that they feel weaker or that they are tripping more frequently. When the hands are affected, all activities of daily living may be affected. It is important to note that regardless of the strength present, loss of sensation will markedly affect function making it difficult to walk, button a shirt, make a phone call, write a letter, etc. Peripheral neuropathies are commonly seen in diabetics and individuals who drink alcohol excessively. There are many other medical conditions that are associated with peripheral neuropathy as well. A good history should include asking about symptoms in family members, as some neuropathies are hereditary.

On physical examination, the patient may have findings consistent with the specific type of neuropathy. For example, a patient with a motor axonal neuropathy may have weakness in the distal muscles with decreased deep tendon reflexes. Patients with a predominantly sensory neuropathy may have diminished sensation to light touch, pinprick, temperature and vibration. If the feet and hands are predominantly affected, the patient is referred to as having a 'stocking–glove' distribution of symptoms. It is important to remember that many patients have a neuropathy that may affect *both* sensory and motor fibers or that affect *both* the axon and the myelin.

Anatomy

Peripheral neuropathies are classified as affecting primarily motor fibers, sensory fibers, or both. They are also classified as to what part of the nerve is predominantly affected – axon, myelin, or both (Fig. 16.1). Finally, neuropathies are classified as segmental (affecting only certain areas of the nerve) or uniform (affecting the entire length of the nerve). Most neuropathies affect the distal segment of the nerve more than the proximal segment. Therefore the longer the nerve, the more it is usually affected. This explains the predominance of findings in the feet in patients with neuropathy.

Table 16.1 Polyneuropathy

EMG finding:	Uniform demyelinating mixed sensorimotor polyneuropathy	Segmental demyelinating meter > sensory polyneuropathy	Axon loss motor > sensory polyneuropathy	Sensory axon loss neuropathy	Axon loss mixed sensorimotor polyneuropathy	Mixed axonal loss & demyelinating sensorimotor polyneuropathy
CMAP amplitude	Normal	Decreased secondary to dispersion or conduction block	Decreased	Normal	Decreased	Decreased
Motor latency	Increased	Increased	Normal	Normal	Normal	Increased
Motor conduction velocity	Decreased	Decreased	Normal	Normal	Normal	Decreased
Dispersion of CMAP	No	Yes	No	No	No	Yes (mild)
SNAP amplitude	Normal	Normal or decreased	Decreased (usually)	Decreased	Decreased	Decreased
SNAP conduction velocity	Decreased	Decreased (somewhat)	Normal	Normal	Normal	Decreased
Needle EMG Would fibs* & PSWs** likely be noted?	No (Normal)	No (Normal)	Yes	No (Normal)	Yes	Yes

Table 16.1 Polyneuropathy (cont'd)

EMG finding:	Uniform demyelinating mixed sensorimotor polyneuropathy	Segmental demyelinating polyneuropathy	Axon loss motor > sensory polyneuropathy	Sensory axon loss neuropathy	Axon loss mixed sensorimotor polyneuropathy	Mixed axonal loss & demyelinating sensorimotor polyneuropathy
Common diseases	1. Hereditary motor sensory neuropathy type I, III, VI (distal weakness with little atrophy) 2. Metachromatic leukodystrophy 3. Krabbe's leukodystrophy 4. Adrenomyelo-neuropathy 5. Congenital hypomyelinating neuropathy 6. Tangier disease 7. Cockayne's syndrome 8. Cerebrotendinous xanthomatosis	1. AIDP†: Guillain–Barré syndrome (ascending proximal weakness) 2. CIDP‡ (weakness of asymmetric low extremities) 3. Osteosclerotic myeloma 4. Leprosy 5. Acute arsenic polyneuropathy 6. Pharmaceuticals (Amiodarone Perhexiline) High dose Ara-C Carcinoma, AIDS	1. Paraneoplastic motor neuronopathy (distal weakness) 2. Porphyria 3. Axonal Guillain–Barré syndrome 4. Hereditary motor sensory neuropathy types II and V 5. Lead neuropathy 6. Dapsone neuropathy	1. Paraneoplastic (sensory, painful in distal extremities) 2. Hereditary sensory neuropathy types I–IV 3. Friedreich's ataxia 4. Spinocerebellar degeneration 5. Abetalipo-proteinemia (Bassen–Kornzweig disease) 6. Primary biliary cirrhosis 7. Acute sensory neuronopathy Cis-platinum toxicity 8. Lymphomatous sensory	1. Alcoholic polyneuropathy (distal symmetric weakness) 2. Vitamin (thiamine, B12) deficiency (distal symmetric weakness) 3. Gouty neuropathy 4. Metal neuropathy (mercury, thallium, gold, etc.) 5. Sarcoidosis 6. Connective tissue diseases (rheumatoid arthritis, SLE, etc.) 7. Gastrectomy, gastric restriction surgery for obesity 8. Chronic liver disease neuropathy of chronic illness 9. Hypothyroidism 10. Myotonic dystrophy 11. AIDS 12. Lyme disease 13. Vincristine neuropathy.	1. Diabetic polyneuropathy (distal symmetric weakness) 2. Uremia (distal symmetric weakness)

Table 16.1 Polyneuropathy (cont'd)

EMG finding:	Uniform demyelinating mixed sensorimotor polyneuropathy	Segmental demyelinating motor > sensory polyneuropathy	Axon loss motor > sensory polyneuropathy	Sensory axon loss neuropathy	Axon loss mixed sensorimotor polyneuropathy	Mixed axonal Loss & demyelinating sensorimotor polyneuropathy
				neuronopathy Chronic idiopathic ataxic neuropathy 9. Sjögren's syndrome 10. Fisher variant Guillain–Barré syndrome 11. Paraproteinemias 12. Pyridoxine toxicity 13. Amyloidosis	etc. 14. Toxic neuropathy (acrylamide, carbon disulfide, carbon monoxide)	

*fibs:fibrillation potentials.
**PSWs: positive sharp waves.
†AIDP: acute inflammatory demyelinating polyneuropathy.
‡CIDP: chronic inflammatory demyelinating polyneuropathy.

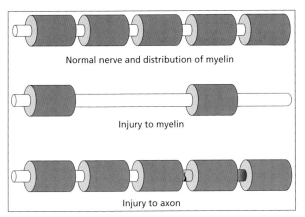

Figure 16.1
Classification of peripheral neuropathies.

 ## Electrodiagnostic Findings

In order to adequately assess for a peripheral neuropathy, sensory and motor nerves must be tested in at least two extremities. Since temperature can affect latency, amplitude and conduction velocity (see Chapter 8, Pitfalls), limb temperature should be maintained at 32°C for the upper extremities and 30°C for the lower extremities. Table 16.1 will help you identify the type of neuropathy based on the electrodiagnostic findings.

Sensory Nerve Conduction Studies

If a peripheral neuropathy involves the sensory fibers, sensory nerve action potentials (SNAPs) may be reduced. If the sensory neuropathy is axonal in nature, the amplitude of the SNAP will be affected, or the response may be unobtainable. If the sensory neuropathy is demyelinating, the SNAP responses can have a decreased conduction velocity. A profound demyelinating process can also result in the loss of SNAPs.

Motor Nerve Conduction Studies

If a peripheral neuropathy involves motor fibers, the compound motor action potential (CMAP) may be affected. If the motor neuropathy is axonal in nature, the amplitude of the CMAP may be affected, or it may be unobtainable. If the motor neuropathy is demyelinating, the CMAP response may have an increased distal latency and/or slowed conduction velocity. Conduction velocity less than 80% of the lower limit of normal suggests a demyelinating neuropathy.

It should be noted whether conduction velocity slowing is uniform throughout the nerve (uniform demyelination), or only affects certain segments of the nerve (segmental demyelination). In segmental demyelination, some of the fibers are traveling slower than other fibers. The CMAP that is generated will be dispersed, meaning it will have a longer duration and lower amplitude (temporal dispersion) (see Fig. 6.1).

When performing motor studies on the peroneal nerve, the active electrode is over the extensor digitorum brevis (EDB) muscle. In many normal people, this muscle is atrophied. Therefore, if the CMAP amplitude is decreased on stimulation of the peroneal nerve with pickup over the EDB, try moving the active electrode to the tibialis anterior muscle. If the amplitude is still low, the findings are significant (i.e., indicate axonal loss).

If the amplitude is decreased in the EDB bilaterally, together with the abductor hallucis, this indicates an axonal peripheral neuropathy.

Late Responses

Since late responses (F-waves and H-reflexes) assess the peripheral nerve along its entire course, these responses are usually affected in peripheral neuropathy. In diseases such as Guillain–Barré syndrome, F-waves can be the earliest indication of a problem, since the proximal segment of the nerve is tested. It should be remembered, however, that these responses are not specific. Therefore, the information generated can help, but not make, the diagnosis.

EMG

EMG findings are usually negative in peripheral neuropathy, unless an axonal motor neuropathy is present. In such cases, affected muscles may demonstrate spontaneous activity (fibrillation potentials and positive sharp waves). Complex repetitive discharges (CRDs) may be noted in chronic neurogenic disorders. Both proximal and distal muscles should be tested. EMG testing is helpful, even when negative, as it helps to rule out other disorders, such as a focal neuropathy or myopathy. In addition, if an axonal lesion is present, the time course of the disease can be assessed by evaluating for the presence of chronic changes in the motor unit action potentials (MUAPs) such as increased duration, polyphasicity or large amplitude (see Chapter 5, Electromyography).

 # Summary

In summary, electrodiagnostic findings in peripheral neuropathy may include:

1. decreased latency and/or conduction velocity in demyelinating neuropathies (decreaed motor latency and/or conduction velocity in motor demyelinating neuropathies and decreased sensory latency and/or conduction velocity in sensory demyelinating neuropathies)
2. decreased amplitude of the CMAP or SNAP in axonal neuropathies (decreasedd CMAP amplitude in motor axonal neuropathies and decreased SNAP amplitudes in sensory axonal neuropathies)
3. abnormal spontaneous activity may be found on needle study in motor axonal neuropathies

See Table 16.1 for a summary of NCS/EMG findings in peripheral neuropathy.

17

Myopathy

Julie Silver

 Clinical Presentation

A myopathy is simply a disorder of the muscles. This can take various forms and the common myopathic disorders are listed in Table 17.1. The primary symptom in myopathies is *weakness*. It is important to note that most myopathies affect the *proximal*

Table 17.1 Common myopathic disorders

Congenital
Centronuclear myopathy
Myotubular myopathy
Nemaline rod myopathy
Fiber-type disproportion
Inflammatory
Polymyositis
Dermatomyositis
Inclusion body myositis
Viral myopathy (e.g., HIV associated myopathy/polymyositis and human T-cell lymphotropic virus-I myopathy)
Sarcoid myopathy
Infectious
Trichinosis
Atrophic
Toxic
Colchicine, azidothymidine (AZT), alcohol, chloroquine, hydroxychloroquine, pentazocine, clofibrate, steroids
Endocrine
Thyroid myopathy
Parathyroid myopathy
Adrenal/steroid myopathy
Pituitary myopathy
Metabolic
Acid maltase deficiency myopathy
Carnitine deficiency myopathy
Debrancher deficiency myopathy
Dystrophies
Dystrophin deficiency (Duchenne and Becker's)
Facioscapulohumeral muscular dystrophy
Myotonic muscular dystrophy
Emery–Dreifuss muscular dystrophy
Oculopharyngeal muscular dystrophy
Limb girdle muscular dystrophy

muscles more than the distal muscles. This means that the first symptom a patient may complain about is difficulty rising from a chair or walking up stairs.

The weakness is *constant* but may be more noticeable when someone is fatigued. In conditions where distal weakness is more prominent (e.g., hereditary distal myopathies) patients may complain of foot drop, unstable ankles, difficulty opening jars or carrying an object in the hand, etc. Pain, when present, is usually not well localized and is an aching or cramping feeling.

Myopathies present as *pure motor conditions*, so the classic presentation is weakness without sensory symptoms. On physical examination it is important to assess strength and muscle atrophy. Most myopathies present with *symmetrical proximal weakness*. In some myopathies, ocular and bulbar muscles are affected, and this should be noted if present. Sensation should be normal and reflexes become increasingly diminished as weakness progresses. Contractures of the joints may develop due to loss of strength.

The usual tests ordered to confirm the diagnosis of myopathy include creatine kinase (CK) serum levels (typically elevated), EMG and muscle biopsy.

Classification

Myopathies can be generally classified as congenital, inflammatory, metabolic, atrophic, or muscular dystrophies (Table 17.1).

Congenital myopathies. Congenital myopathies typically present in the first few years of life, but occasionally there are people who are diagnosed as an adult. The clinical symptoms are usually non-specific. Most of the myopathies in this category have fairly typical histochemical findings when stained, so muscle biopsy is generally needed to confirm the diagnosis.

Inflammatory myopathies. Most inflammatory myopathies are presumably due to some type of immunologic attack of the muscles. However, there are some inflammatory myopathies that are known to be due to infection caused by parasites, viruses or bacteria.

Metabolic myopathies. These are caused by inherited enzyme deficiencies that are essential for intracellular energy production. These may present as a typical non-specific myopathy with proximal weakness as the only clue, or with cramps and myoglobinuria. In some cases metabolic myopathies are part of a more diffuse neurologic syndrome that may involve the central nervous system (CNS). Patients may become symptomatic only after exercise. CK levels are typically very elevated.

Muscular dystrophies. These are inherited muscular disorders, often with an early onset and very progressive course. Some muscular dystrophies can now be identified by a specific chromosomal abnormality or gene product (e.g., Duchenne and Becker's dystrophy).

Electrodiagnostic Findings

EMG plays an important role in the diagnosis of myopathy and is frequently done in conjunction with a muscle biopsy. EMG not only helps to determine the diagnosis and extent of the disease, but can also be an important indicator of where the muscle biopsy should be obtained.

Some electrodiagnosticians perform just the EMG portion of the test if myopathy is the suspected diagnosis, because the nerve conduction studies should be *normal*. However, if there is a concurrent neuropathy, this likely will be missed with only EMG studies. So, it is useful to perform at least one motor and one sensory nerve conduction study as a screen when testing for myopathy.

Sensory Nerve Conduction Studies

Sensory nerve conduction studies should be normal in patients with myopathy.

Motor Nerve Conduction Studies

Motor nerve conduction studies are typically normal in myopathy, since the active electrode is usually over a *distal* muscle. However, if the myopathy is severe enough to affect both distal and proximal muscles or is one of the less common myopathies that preferentially affect distal muscles, then the motor nerve conduction studies may be abnormal. In these cases there may be evidence of reduced compound muscle action potential (CMAP) amplitude. The distal latencies and conduction velocities will be normal, as the myelin is not affected.

Late Responses

Late responses are not usually helpful in myopathies as they are non-specific.

EMG

Myopathies present with characteristic findings on EMG. Myopathic motor units are usually of short duration, small amplitude, polyphasic and have early recruitment (see Fig. 5.14). This would be seen as a large number of small motor units firing for a minimal contraction. The motor unit action potential (MUAP) is typically smaller due to dropout or dysfunction of individual muscle fibers. This leads to a decreased size of the motor unit. The number of motor units usually remains the same except in severe cases where every single fiber drops out and thus eliminates that motor unit.

Spontaneous activity is frequently noted in myopathies. Many myopathies present with positive sharp waves and fibrillation potentials (fibs). Less commonly myopathies may reveal *myotonic discharges* (see Chapter 5, Electromyography). It is not uncommon in chronic myopathies to note *complex repetitive discharges* (CRDs). Rarely there is evidence of *contracture,* which is the *complete absence of electrical activity in the contracted state.*

The EMG study should first focus on the weakest muscles. Typically these are the more proximal muscles. In some instances, the only abnormalities may be in the paraspinal muscles. If these show the typical findings consistent with myopathy, then stronger muscles should be tested as well in order to determine the extent of the disease. If the clinically weakest muscles are normal, then testing the stronger muscles will not be useful and is not advised. In cases where the muscles show neuropathic instead of myopathic changes, the electromyographer needs to reconsider the scope of the study and expand it to rule out other conditions. In this instance, nerve conduction testing would definitely be indicated. It should also be noted that steroid myopathies predominantly affect Type II fibers. Since EMG testing evaluates Type I fibers, EMG testing is often normal in steroid myopathy.

There are three additional considerations when performing an EMG in a suspected myopathic patient. First, it is not a good idea to order a CK blood test shortly after the EMG as the levels may be falsely elevated. Second, when determining which muscle to biopsy it is wise to choose a muscle that is affected but not completely atrophic. Third, do not test all affected muscles, because once they have been needled, they should not be used for a biopsy. The EMG report should clearly identify which muscles have not been tested so that an appropriate decision can be made for which muscle to biopsy.

Summary

In summary, electrodiagnostic findings in myopathy may include:

1. normal SNAP
2. normal CMAP
3. spontaneous potentials (PSWs and fibs) in affected muscles
4. short duration small amplitude polyphasic motor units with early recruitment in affected muscles on EMG.

18

Brachial Plexopathies

Walter Gaudino

 ## Clinical Presentation

Evaluation of the brachial plexus is one of the most challenging examinations that the electromyographer will encounter. This is due to the complexity of the anatomy and its relative inaccessibility. Moreover, standard nerve conduction protocols do not test many parts of the brachial plexus. A thorough understanding of the anatomy of the brachial plexus is integral to performing an accurate electrodiagnostic study.

Clinical presentations vary according to the area of the brachial plexus that is involved. Most brachial plexus lesions are due to trauma, either obstetrical or accidental e.g., motor vehicle, knife or projectile injuries. The majority of brachial plexus lesions in adults are unilateral and affect the dominant limb more commonly than the non-dominant limb. Obstetric palsies affect the right side more than the left. The history and physical examination varies with the type of lesion to the brachial plexus. One useful way to classify the varied brachial plexus lesions is on the basis of their anatomic location. Brachial plexus lesions can be classified into supraclavicular, infraclavicular and pan plexus lesions (Table 18.1).

The clinical presentation of the lesions of the brachial plexus varies according to the site of the brachial plexus involved. Injuries to the lateral cord may present with numbness in the lateral aspect of the forearm below the elbow extending just above the thumb. This is the distribution of the *lateral cutaneous nerve of the forearm*. This may be associated with numbness in the distribution of the median nerve (the 1st, 2nd and 3rd digits), and weakness of the biceps, brachioradialis and pronator teres muscles. A lesion affecting the medial cord may damage the *medial antebrachial cutaneous nerve* and present with

Table 18.1 Brachial plexus lesions

Supraclavicular	Infraclavicular	Pan plexus
Roots/upper trunks	Radiation related	Trauma
Incomplete traction injury	Gunshot wound	Severe traction injury
Erb's palsy	Humeral fracture/dislocation	Late metastatic disease
C5, C6 root avulsions	Dislocation	Late radiation palsy
Axillary nerve block		
Lower plexus		
(Roots/lower trunk)		
Metastatic tumor		
Pancoast syndrome		
Post sternotomy		
Thoracic outlet syndrome		
Klumpke's palsy (C8, T1)		

Figure 18.1
Cutaneous
innervation.

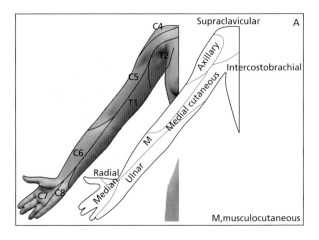

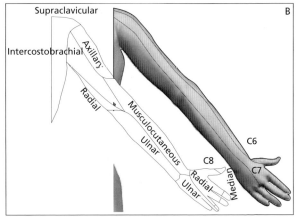

numbness of the medial aspect of the forearm. This may be associated with weakness of the flexor carpi ulnaris (FCU), abductor pollicis brevis (APB), opponens pollicis, flexor digitorum indicis (FDI), abductor digit minimi (ADM), and adductor pollicis muscles.

Brachial plexopathy due to carcinomatous spread usually presents with *pain.* These lesions may present as a result of spread from an adjacent breast or lung mass. These plexopathies have a predilection for the lower trunks, but can also involve a more diffuse pattern. Brachial plexopathy may develop from months to years after radiation treatment of breast, lung, and mediastinal cancer. These plexopathies typically are not painful, but present with paresthesias and sensory loss that progress slowly. They tend to be more prominent in the upper trunk distribution. Figures 18.1 and 18.2 review the cutaneous innervation of the extremities.

 Anatomy

The brachial plexus (Fig. 18.3) is an intricate neural web that provides the innervation to the neck and the upper extremities. Most commonly the plexus arises from the anterior

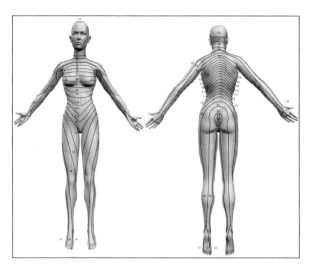

Figure 18.2
Cutaneous
innervation.

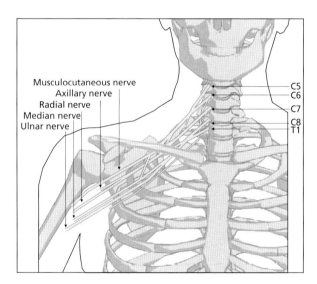

Figure 18.3 The
brachial plexus.

Musculocutaneous nerve
Axillary nerve
Radial nerve
Median nerve
Ulnar nerve

C5
C6
C7
C8
T1

rami of the C5 through the T1 nerves. There are variants on the theme with some patients having contributions from the C4 level or the T2 levels. These are known as pre-fixed and post-fixed plexi respectively. The following discussion will focus on the most common pattern of innervation (i.e., C5 to T1).

There are many methods to help learn the anatomy of the plexus. The anatomy need not be intimidating. You can remember the section of the brachial plexus using the mnemonic 'Robert Taylor Drinks Coors Beer' along with three parallel lines; an X, a Y and an M. The mnemonic stands for the five sections of the brachial plexus, which are the roots, trunks, divisions, cords, and branches.

Figure 18.4 The
roots of the
brachial plexus.

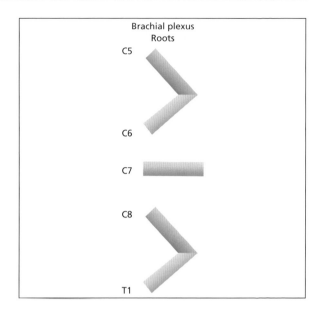

Figure 18.5 The
structure of the
brachial plexus.

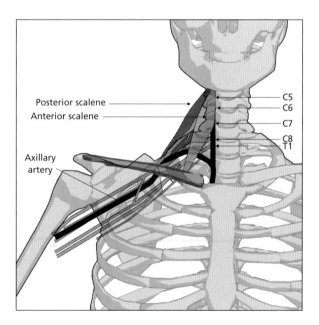

Start the drawing of the brachial plexus by representing the C5–T1 nerve roots by
five down-sloping horizontal lines and label them C5, C6, C7, C8, and T1. The *roots* of
the plexus originate at the anterior rami of C5 through the T1 nerves (Fig. 18.4). The
roots run through the anterior and posterior scalene muscles (Fig. 18.5). It is at this level
that the C5 and C6 roots converge to form the upper trunk, the C7 root forms the middle

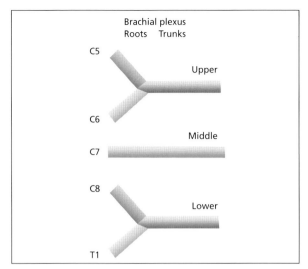

Figure 18.6 The structure of the brachial plexus.

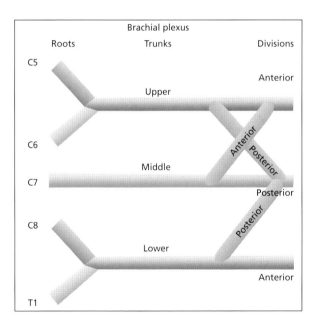

Figure 18.7 The structure of the brachial plexus.

trunk and the C8 and T1 roots form the *lower trunk*. Then connect the roots to the three parallel lines as in Figure 18.6. These represent the roots and the trunks of the brachial plexus.

The trunks slope down and divide to form the *anterior and posterior divisions* (Fig. 18.7). The divisions are found deep under the middle section of the clavicle. They run along a parallel course to the subclavian artery. They then weave around the axillary artery. At this point the posterior divisions of the upper and lower trunks join the middle trunk to form the posterior cord. The anterior division of the middle trunk joins the upper trunk fibers to become the lateral cord. At this level the brachial plexus is divided into *lateral, posterior and medial cords* that are named in their relationship to the axillary artery (Fig. 18.8). The brachial plexus then goes on to divide into the terminal nerve branches (Fig. 18.9). The posterior cord becomes the radial nerve, but also gives off the axillary nerve. The lateral cord terminates in the *musculocutaneous nerve* as well as a branch that merges with a branch from the medial cord to form the *median nerve*. The medial cord and terminates in the ulnar nerve.

Along its course, the brachial plexus gives off *collateral* nerves. These nerves are helpful in that they can be used to help localize lesions either proximal or distal to the brachial plexus. Some of the clinically more important nerves include the *dorsal scapular nerve* to the rhomboids (involvement will localize the lesion above the level of the trunks). The *suprascapular nerve* to the supraspinatus and infraspinatus comes off at the trunk level. For example, plexopathies involving the upper trunk can usually be distinguished

Figure 18.8 The structure of the brachial plexus.

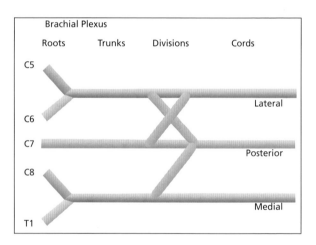

Figure 18.9 The structure of the brachial plexus.

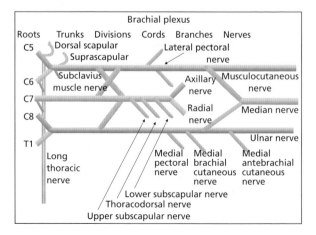

from lesions of the lateral cord. Although both will have reduced amplitudes of the musculocutaneous compound muscle action potentials (CMAPs), *lateral antebrachial* sensory nerve action potential (SNAP), and *median* SNAP, only the upper trunk lesion will have a decreased amplitude of the *axillary nerve* CMAP recorded from the deltoid muscle and *suprascapular* CMAP recorded from supraspinatus muscle. Only the upper trunk lesion may have spontaneous potentials in the deltoid, brachial radialis, infraspinatus, or supraspinatus muscles. These relationships will be further reviewed in the next section.

 Electrodiagnosis

A properly planned and technically correct brachial plexus electrodiagnostic examination can give more information than a physical examination alone. The electrodiagnostic examination is the most sensitive physiologic examination of the brachial plexus. This test can help to localize the site of the lesion *and* provide the electromyographer with an estimate of the prognosis of the lesion. When performing an examination to rule out a brachial plexus lesion it is important to use the unaffected limb as a control and compare nerve responses from the two sides tested.

Examination of the brachial plexus will require learning many non-standard nerve tests. Standard ulnar and median motor and sensory nerve evaluation examines only the medial cord and lower trunk. Median sensory nerve studies are testing the upper trunk or lateral cord. A brachial plexus lesion is proximal to the segments of these nerves that are being tested. Extensive electromyography is essential to localize the area of the brachial plexus that is affected, and to rule out possible radiculopathies and mononeuropathies as the source of the patient's symptoms.

Aside from localizing the lesion, the electrodiagnostic test can also establish the severity of nerve damage. Axon loss plexopathy is the most likely type of pattern seen in the electrodiagnostic lab. The electrophysiologic changes depend upon the severity of the axonal loss.

Sensory Nerve Conduction Studies

The sensory nerve conduction study is a more sensitive indicator of injury to the brachial plexus than the motor nerve response. The sensory nerve distal latency and conduction velocity are usually normal in brachial plexus lesions. This is because the lesion is usually axonal. However, the sensory nerve action potential amplitude (SNAP) may be decreased in lesions affecting the brachial plexus. With mild lesions of the brachial plexus the SNAP amplitude may be unaffected. With increasing severity of injury to the brachial plexus the amplitude of the appropriate SNAP may be decreased or absent. The SNAP amplitude reflects the number of functioning axons in continuity with the sensory root cell body. This is also called the dorsal root ganglion (Fig. 18.10). Lesions that are proximal to this cell body, such as radiculopathies and nerve root avulsions, do not interfere with the function of the cell body on the sensory nerves derived from that root. Therefore lesions *proximal* to the dorsal root ganglion have intact sensory nerve electrical function, even though sensation may be affected clinically.

Lesions *proximal* to the dorsal root ganglion have a normal SNAP amplitude. Lesions *distal* to the dorsal root ganglion *disconnect the sensory nerve cell body from its axons*. This results in deprivation of the axons from their nutritional source. Depending on the severity of the lesion this may result in a decrement or absence of the SNAP potential. *The differentiation between pre- and postganglionic lesions is extremely important.* Although

Figure 18.10 SNAP amplitude may be decreased in lesions affecting the brachial plexus.

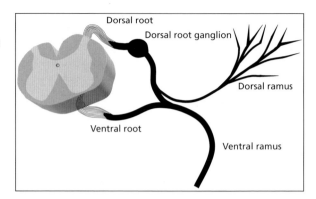

both lesions may present with numbness and sensory loss in a defined distribution, the nerve root avulsion (preganglionic lesion) usually portends a dismal prognosis. Such injuries do not undergo spontaneous regeneration and are poorly amenable to surgical repair. The postganglionic lesions have a much more favorable prognosis.

Motor Nerve Conduction Studies

The compound muscle action potential amplitudes (CMAP) are not affected unless the brachial plexus injury is severe. With severe injuries to the brachial plexus there may be a reduction in the appropriate CMAP amplitudes. When they are affected, the CMAP is generally a better indication of the extent of axonal loss than SNAP amplitudes. When looking for a decrease in the amplitude, consider the nerve you are testing and the level affected in the brachial plexus. (CMAPs from ADM and APB should be equally reduced.)

Stimulating at Erb's point may reveal decreased amplitude if a conduction block is present distal to that point. The motor latencies and conduction velocities are usually unaffected by a brachial plexus lesion because they are a function of the fibers that are intact and do not reflect abnormal conduction across the brachial plexus. However, stimulation across Erb's point may reveal slowing if there is a demyelinating lesion in the brachial plexus.

Late Responses

Most lesions of the brachial plexus are incomplete and have normal conduction across the brachial plexus. The lesion may be so localized that the effect of the lesion is 'diluted' along the neural path of transmission of the F-wave. Therefore, F-wave prolongation is a non-specific finding.

EMG

Your findings on the history and physical examination will help you decide which muscles to examine electromyographically. The EMG testing should be mapped out based on a review of the brachial plexus (Fig. 18.9) before the test is started. Electrodiagnostic findings with acute mild plexopathies are usually limited to fibrillations and positive sharp waves in an appropriate pattern. For example, a lesion of the lateral cord may have positive sharp waves noted in the biceps, pronator teres, flexor carpi radialis (FCR) and the pectoralis muscles. The supraspinatus, infraspinatus and levator scapulae muscles would

Table 18.2 Localization of lesions in the brachial plexus

Anatomical area of Injury	Affected sensory NCS	Affected motor NCS	Positive findings EMG
Radiculopathy	Normal	CMAPs decreased	Cervical paraspinals Myotomal pattern
Upper trunk	Lateral antebrachial Median nerve to 1st digit Radial	Musculocutaneous nerve to biceps Suprascapular nerve to supraspinatus Axillary nerve to deltoid	Supraspinatus Biceps Pronator teres Deltoid Brachial radialis
Middle trunk	Median nerve to 3rd digit and 4th digit	Radial nerve to extensor digitorum communis	Latissimus dorsi Teres major Extensor digitorum communis Pronator teres Flexor carpi radialis
Lower trunk	Ulnar nerve to 5th digit Medial antebrachial	Ulnar nerve to abductor digiti minimi Median nerve to abductor pollicis brevis	Flexor digitorum superficialis Abductor digitorum minimi Flexor carpi ulnaris Flexor superficialis Flexor digitorum profundus
Lateral cord	Lateral antebrachial Median nerve to 1st digit	Musculocutaneous nerve to biceps	Biceps Pronator teres Flexor carpi radialis
Posterior cord	Radial	Axillary nerve to deltoid Radial nerve to extensor carpi ulnaris	Latissimus dorsi Teres major Deltoid Radial muscles
Medial cord	Ulnar nerve to 5th digit Medial antebrachial nerve	Ulnar nerve to abductor digiti minimi Median nerve to abductor pollicis brevis	Ulnar muscles Flexor digitorum superficialis Flexor pollicis longus Abductor pollicis brevis

be normal. In lesions where reinnervation has occurred, long duration, high amplitude or polyphasicity may be noted in the MUAPs.

The clinical manifestations of an injury to the brachial plexus are maximal at onset but the electrodiagnostic findings may take up to three weeks to develop. *It is important that the electrodiagnostic test be delayed three weeks after the onset of the injury,* so that sufficient Wallerian degeneration of the distal parts of the injured nerves can occur. This allows for the development of fibrillation potentials and positive sharp waves. Testing prior to that time frame may yield confusing and misleading data. Cervical paraspinals are expected to be *normal* in brachial plexus lesions because the paraspinal muscles are innervated by the posterior rami and the brachial plexus is innervated by the anterior rami of the spinal nerve. Table 18.2 maps out the electrodiagnosis of the brachial plexus.

By reviewing the table, you can localize the lesions to the roots or areas of the brachial plexus.

Summary

In summary, the electrodiagnostic findings in brachial plexopathy may include (see Table 18.2):

1. Decreased SNAP amplitude
2. Decreased CMAP amplitude
3. Slowing of conduction velocity with stimulation across Erb's point
4. Normal EMG findings in the paraspinal muscles
5. Spontaneous activity (fibs and PSWs) in muscles distal to the level of the injury.

19

Lumbosacral Plexopathies

Walter Gaudino

Electrodiagnostic evaluations of the lumbar and sacral plexus (LSP) can be challenging examinations. This is due to the complexity of the anatomy and its relative inaccessibility. Moreover, standard nerve conduction protocols do not test many parts of these areas. A thorough understanding of the anatomy is integral to performing an accurate electrodiagnostic study.

Clinical Presentation

Neurologic damage to the lumbar and sacral plexus is less common than in the brachial plexus. This is due to the relatively protected position of these neural structures and their decreased accessibility to injury. Lumbosacral plexopathies can be caused by anatomic injury and abnormalities, such as tumors, hematomas, surgical damage and trauma. The LSP can also be damaged by metabolic insults such as diabetes mellitus, infection, vasculitis, or paraneoplastic syndromes. The presentation of the plexopathy varies according to the structures involved.

Anatomy

The anatomy of the lumbar and sacral plexi will be discussed separately. The lumbar plexus (Fig. 19.1) is an intricate neural web that provides innervations to the abdominal

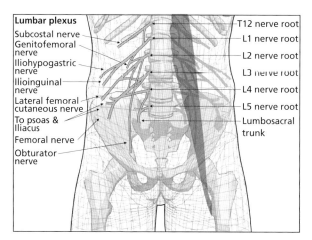

Figure 19.1
Anatomy of the lumbar plexus.

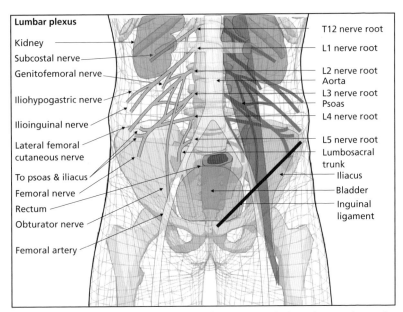

Lumbar plexus

Kidney
Subcostal nerve
Genitofemoral nerve
Iliohypogastric nerve
Ilioinguinal nerve
Lateral femoral cutaneous nerve
To psoas & iliacus
Femoral nerve
Rectum
Obturator nerve
Femoral artery

T12 nerve root
L1 nerve root
L2 nerve root
Aorta
L3 nerve root
Psoas
L4 nerve root
L5 nerve root
Lumbosacral trunk
Iliacus
Bladder
Inguinal ligament

Figure 19.2 The lumbar plexus is formed in the psoas muscle from the anterior rami of the upper four lumbar nerves L1, L2, L3 and L4.

wall and the anterior-medial aspect of the thigh. The lumbar plexus is formed in the psoas muscle from the anterior rami of the upper four lumbar nerves L1, L2, L3 and L4. There is sometimes a contribution from T12, but this is variable. The branches of the plexus emerge from the lateral, medial and anterior borders of the muscle. The *iliohypogastric, ilioinguinal, femoral* and *lateral femoral cutaneous nerves* arise from the lateral aspect of the psoas muscle. The *obturator nerve* arises from the medial aspect of the psoas muscle. The *genitofemoral nerve* arises from the anterior aspect of the psoas muscle (Fig. 19.2).

The lumbar plexus has a much simpler pattern than the brachial plexus, because it lacks the distinct subdivisions such as trunks and cords that is characteristic of the brachial plexus. The lumbar plexus consists of anterior primary rami, and these rami divide into *anterior* and *posterior* divisions.

Nerve roots from L1, L2, L3 and L4 transverse through the psoas muscle and then coalesce, to divide into anterior and posterior divisions. The lumbar plexus then terminates into seven major branches. The first three provide motor and sensory innervation to the abdominal wall and groin. These are the *iliohypogastric, ilioinguinal* and *genitofemoral nerves* respectively. The next three go on to innervate the thigh's anterior and medial aspects. These are the *lateral femoral cutaneous, femoral* and *obturator nerves*. The 7th branch is a contribution from L4 to the sacral plexus. The obturator nerves derive from the anterior divisions. The lateral femoral cutaneous and the femoral nerves arise from the posterior divisions. The femoral nerve terminates into the *saphenous nerve* that provides sensation to the medial aspect of the leg. Table 19.1 summarizes the nerves of the lumbar plexus and their respective neural innervation pathways.

The sacral plexus (Figs 19.3 and 19.4) is similar to the lumbar plexus in that it is primarily a collection of ventral primary spinal nerves that divide into anterior and

Table 19.1 The lumbar plexus

Peripheral nerve	Root	Division	Sensation	Muscle
Iliohypogastric	L1,2		Superior gluteal region	None
Genitofemoral	L1,2		Scrotal skin/adjacent thigh and labia	None
Lateral femoral cutaneous	L2,3	Posterior	Anterolateral thigh	None
Femoral	L2,3,4	Posterior	Anterior thigh, anteromedial thigh Medial leg/foot via the saphenous division of the femoral nerve	Sartorious Iliacus Pectinous Quadriceps
Obturator	L2,3,4	Anterior	Medial thigh	Adductor longus, Gracilis Adductor brevis Obturator internus Adductor magnus

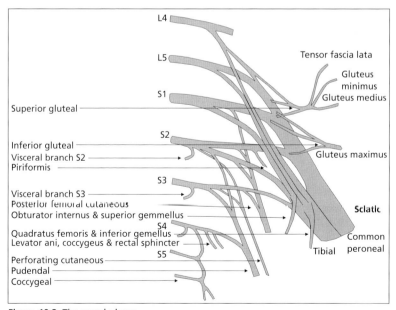

Figure 19.3 The sacral plexus.

Figure 19.4 The plexus is formed in the posterior aspect of the pelvis and lies in the back of the pelvis between the piriformis muscle and the pelvic fascia.

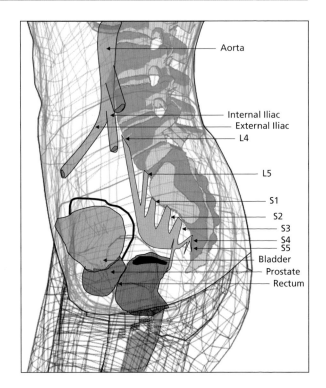

posterior divisions. These, in turn, divide into multiple peripheral nerves. The sacral plexus provides sensation, muscular and articular innervation to the posterior hip girdle, thigh and anterior and posterior leg regions. The sacral plexus is composed of primary ventral rami from the L4–S3 levels. Although the sacral plexus appears intimidating it is actually quite simple to learn. The plexus is formed in the posterior aspect of the pelvis and lies in the back of the pelvis between the piriformis muscle and the pelvic fascia (Fig. 19.4).

In front of the sacral plexus are the hypogastric vessels, the ureter and the sigmoid colon. The superior gluteal and the inferior gluteal vessels run between the 1st, 2nd and 3rd sacral nerves respectively. The close anatomic relationship to these blood vessels makes this structure vulnerable to trauma, which may lead to bleeding.

The sacral plexus is formed from the ventral primary rami from the L4 through the S3 nerves. All of the nerves (except the S3 root) then divide into an anterior and posterior division. The plexus gives off a number of branches, five of which are important to remember for electrodiagnostic testing of this area. The *five essential nerves* are the *superior and inferior gluteal*, the *posterior femoral cutaneous, sciatic* and the *pudendal*. The sciatic nerve divides into the common peroneal and tibial divisions in the thigh. The gluteal, posterior femoral cutaneous and the common peroneal division of the sciatic nerve arise from the posterior components of the sacral plexus. The tibial division of the sciatic nerve, pudendal and muscular branches to the quadratus femoris, gemellus inferior, obturator internus, and gemellus superior muscles arise from the anterior components of the sacral plexus. Table 19.2 reviews the main contents of the sacral plexus.

Table 19.2 The sacral plexus

Peripheral nerve	Root	Division	Sensation	Muscle
Superior gluteal	L4,5, S1	Posterior	None	Gluteus minimus, & medius Tensor fascia lata
Inferior gluteal	L5, S1,2	Posterior	None	Gluteus maximus
Posterior femoral cutaneous	L2,3,4	Posterior	Posterior thigh, Scrotum/labia Proximal calf, lower border of gluteus maximus	None
Sciatic (peroneal)	L4,5, S1,2	Posterior	Posterolateral leg, web space between 1st and 2nd toes dorsal/medial leg	Short head of biceps Femoris, tibialis anterior Extensor digitorum brevis (EDB) Peroneus tertius, brevis and longus
Sciatic (tibial)	L4,5, S1,2,3	Anterior	Posterior leg, lateral foot, sole foot	Long head of biceps, Semi-membranous, Semitendinosus Adductor magnus, Plantaris, Popliteus, Gastrocnemius, Tibialis posterior Soleus, Flexor digitorum longus, Flexor, hallucis longus

Electrodiagnostic Findings

The electrodiagnostic examination is the most sensitive physiologic examination of the lumbosacral plexus. This test can help to localize the site of the lesion *and* prognosticate. When performing an examination to rule out a lumbar or sacral lesion, it is important to use the unaffected limb as a control and compare nerve responses from the two sides.

Examination of the lumbosacral plexus may necessitate a few non-standard nerve tests. For example, the lumbar plexus may require evaluation of the saphenous portion of the femoral nerve, the lateral femoral cutaneous nerve of the thigh and the femoral nerve. The sacral plexus may require evaluation of the superficial peroneal and sural sensory nerves. The peroneal motor response from both the extensor digitorum brevis and the tibialis anterior muscles may be required. The tibial response may be recorded from the abductor hallucis and the abductor digiti quinti. Extensive needle electromyography is essential to localize the area of the plexus that is affected, and to rule out possible radiculopathies or mononeuropathies as the source of the patient's symptoms. Aside from localizing the lesion, the electrodiagnostic test can also establish the severity of nerve damage.

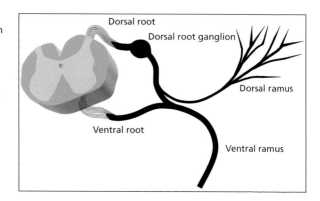

Figure 19.5 In order for an axon to function it must be in contact with the sensory root cell body (also called the dorsal root ganglion).

Dorsal root

Dorsal root ganglion

Dorsal ramus

Ventral root

Ventral ramus

Sensory Nerve Conduction Studies

The sensory nerve is a more sensitive indicator of injury to the plexus than the motor nerve response. The sensory nerve distal latency and conduction velocity are usually *normal* in plexus lesions; however, the sensory nerve action potential (SNAP) amplitude may be *decreased* in lesions affecting the plexus. With mild lesions of the lumbar or sacral plexus, the SNAP amplitude may be unaffected. With increasing severity of injury to the plexus the amplitude of the appropriate SNAPs may be decreased or absent. The SNAP amplitude is a summation of individual functioning sensory axons. In order for an axon to function it must be in contact with the sensory root cell body. This is also called the dorsal root ganglion (Fig. 19.5).

Lesions that are proximal to this cell body, such as radiculopathies and nerve root avulsions, do not interfere with the trophic function of the cell body on the sensory nerves derived from that root. Therefore lesions *proximal* to the dorsal root ganglion have intact sensory nerve electrical function. This results in normal SNAP parameters even in the presence of sensory loss. Lesions *distal* to the dorsal root ganglion disconnect the sensory nerve cell body from its axons. This results in death of the disconnected axons because they are deprived of the nutrition that they need to survive. Depending on the severity of the lesion this may result in a decrement or absence of the SNAP amplitude. The differentiation of preganglionic and postganglionic lesions is extremely important. Although both lesions may present with numbness and sensory loss in a defined distribution, the nerve root avulsion usually portends a poorer prognosis because these injuries do not undergo spontaneous regeneration and are usually not amenable to surgical repair. The postganglionic lesions have a more favorable prognosis.

Motor Nerve Conduction Studies

In general, with lumbosacral plexopathies, the motor latencies and velocities are within normal limits. The compound muscle action potential (CMAP) amplitudes are usually not affected unless the injury is severe. With severe injuries to the plexus there may be a reduction in the amplitude of the corresponding CMAP. As with the brachial plexus, when CMAP amplitudes are affected, they are generally a better indicator of the extent of axonal loss than SNAP abnormalities. Side to side amplitude differences can give an approximation of the degree of axonal injury during the first few months following injury. For example, a 70% decrement in CMAP amplitude roughly correlates to a 70% axon loss. The motor latencies and conduction velocities are usually unaffected by a lumbar or sacral lesion, because they are a function of the fibers that are intact and do not reflect abnormal conduction across the plexus. One should be cautioned that due to normal wear and tear and day-to-day trauma, atrophy of intrinsic foot muscles and side-to-side amplitude differences are not that unusual, even in asymptomatic individuals. For this reason, amplitude differences of less than 50% may not be significant, depending on the clinical picture.

Late Responses

Most lesions of the lumbosacral plexus are incomplete and have many areas of normal conduction across the lumbosacral plexus. The lesion may be so localized that the affect of the lesion is 'diluted' along the neural path of transmission of the H-reflex and F-wave. Therefore, H-reflexes and F-waves are usually *not* helpful in the diagnosis of plexopathies.

EMG

Your findings on the history and physical examination will help guide you in determining which muscles to examine electromyographically. Refer to Tables 19.1 and 19.2 to help design your study. Electrodiagnostic findings in plexopathies may include fibrillations and positive sharp waves in all muscles innervated distal to the lesion. In chronic lesions, motor unit action potentials may demonstrate long duration, high amplitude, and polyphasic potentials. Recruitment is usually decreased in all affected muscles.

The clinical manifestations of an injury to the plexus are apparent at onset but the electromyographic findings may take up to three weeks to develop. It is important that the test be delayed three weeks after the onset of injury so that Wallerian degeneration of the distal parts of the injured nerves occurs – this allows for the development of fibrillation potentials and positive sharp waves. Testing prior to that time-frame can yield confusing and misleading data. Lumbar paraspinals are expected to be normal in lumbar and sacral plexus lesions because the paraspinal muscles are innervated by the posterior rami, and the plexus is innervated by the anterior rami of the spinal nerve.

A classic lumbar plexus injury may have decreased saphenous, femoral and lateral femoral cutaneous amplitudes, with intact latencies and conduction velocities. In addition, EMG would reveal muscle membrane instability in the vastus medialis obliquus, adductor brevis, sartorius and iliopsoas. The lumbar paraspinal muscles would test normal in a pure lumbar plexopathy. By using these guidelines, a thorough electrodiagnostic evaluation of the lumbosacral plexus can be planned and carried out with a minimum of discomfort to the patient.

Summary

In summary, the electrodiagnostic findings in lumbosacral plexopathy may include:

1. Decreased SNAP amplitude
2. Decreased CMAP amplitude
3. Normal EMG findings in the paraspinal mucles
4. Abnormal spontaneous activity (fibs and PSWs) in muscles distal to the level of the injury

20

Motor Neuron Diseases

Lyn Weiss

Motor neuron diseases represent a group of diseases with the primary pathology located in the spinal cord and affecting both upper and/or lower motor neurons. They include poliomyelitis, amyotrophic lateral sclerosis (ALS), progressive muscular atrophy, progressive lateral sclerosis and progressive bulbar palsy. Although many of these diseases affect both upper and lower motor neurons, *only the injury to the lower motor neurons can be assessed with electrodiagnostic testing.*

The diagnosis of motor neuron disease is based on the electrodiagnostic findings in conjunction with the physical examination, neuroimaging, and laboratory studies. The goal of electrodiagnostic studies is to assess for lower motor neuron dysfunction in clinically affected regions as well as in regions that are clinically unaffected.[1] The gravity and significance of a diagnosis of motor neuron disease is of such magnitude that if this diagnosis is suspected, referral to a physician with significant experience in this area is recommended.

 ## Clinical Presentation

Patients with motor neuron diseases typically present with findings of *both* upper and lower motor neuron abnormalities on physical examination. The exceptions to this would be poliomyelitis and progressive muscular atrophy, which affect only the lower motor neurons, and progressive lateral sclerosis, which affects only the upper motor neurons. Signs and symptoms of upper motor neuron involvement may include spasticity, stiffness and impaired motor control. Signs and symptoms of lower motor neuron involvement may include muscle atrophy, weakness, flaccidity, fasciculations and cramps.

 ## Anatomy

As stated above, motor neuron diseases can affect either the upper and/or the lower motor neuron. These disorders are specific for the motor system affecting the motor cortex, corticospinal (motor) tracts and the anterior horn cells. There is usually no significant sensory or cognitive effect.

 ## Electrodiagnostic Findings

Sensory Nerve Conduction Studies

Because motor neuron diseases affect the anterior horn cell and not the dorsal root ganglion, sensory nerve action potentials should show *normal* amplitude and conduction velocities.

Motor Nerve Conduction Studies

Compound muscle action potential (CMAP) latencies and conduction velocities should be normal, as the myelin is intact. Because of axon loss, the amplitude of the CMAPs may be markedly reduced. If there is severe axonal loss, some of the fastest fibers may be lost. Therefore, one may see *mildly* increased latency and decreased conduction velocity, but the amount of slowing should not exceed about 20% of normal.

Late Responses

F-waves and H-reflexes are generally not helpful in the diagnosis of motor neuron disease as they are non-specific, however they can be beneficial in ruling out other diagnoses.

 # EMG

In order to diagnose a disease of the anterior horn cells, three limbs, or two limbs and bulbar muscles should show spontaneous potentials (fibs or positive sharp waves). Both proximal and distal muscles corresponding to various myotomal distributions should be tested. Fasciculation potentials as well as complex repetitive discharges (CRDs) may be observed. Motor unit action potentials (MUAPs) may be of long duration, increased polyphasicity and large amplitude, indicating reinnervation. Decreased recruitment should be noted.

 # Summary

The electrodiagnostic findings in motor neuron diseases may include the following:

1. Normal SNAP amplitude and conduction velocity.
2. CMAPs have decreased amplitude with normal (or mildly increased) latency and normal (or mildly decreased) conduction velocity.
3. EMG will demonstrate spontaneous potentials (fibs and PSWs) in affected muscles. Fasciculations and CRDs may also be noted. MUAPs may show increased duration, large amplitude polyphasic potentials if reinnervation has occurred. There will be decreased recruitment as well. Remember to test at least three limbs, or two limbs and bulbar muscles.

REFERENCE
1. Misulis K. Essentials of Clinical Neurophysiology. London: Butterworth-Heinemann, 1997.

21

How to Write a Report

Lyn Weiss

Writing a meaningful report will help convey your findings to the referring physician. Most reports contain the following information:

1. Patient's name, identification number (if applicable), date of test, name of physician performing the test, and referring physician.
2. Brief history and physical.
3. Table of findings (usually printed out from the tabular data). This is important in case the test needs to be repeated at a later date. Results can be compared for electrophysiological improvement or progression.
4. Findings. The pertinent findings should be discussed. Specific nerve or muscle abnormalities can be discussed.
5. Conclusion. The conclusion should be written with the referring physician's reason for the testing kept in mind.

Findings

For each motor nerve tested, the latency, amplitude (and/or area under the curve) and conduction velocity should be reported. Since the tabular data is usually included as part of the report, specific numbers are usually not necessary in this section of the report. It is helpful if the tabular printout flags abnormal values or alternatively labels individual nerves as increased, decreased or normal. Abnormal findings should be highlighted in this area. Abnormalities can be recorded as increased or decreased. In instances of severe abnormalities, when a number is far outside the normal range, (i.e. median distal motor latency of 8.2 msec or an amplitude decrement of 80%) it would be appropriate to mention it.

For each *sensory* nerve tested, *amplitude* and distal latency or *conduction velocity* should be recorded. Once again, if this is a tabular printout these do not need to be listed again. Abnormalities, however, should be noted. These can be reported as *increased, decreased, or normal*. Note that since the sensory response contains no myoneural junction, the latency reflects the conduction velocity. In motor nerves, this myoneural junction must be 'factored out' by obtaining two latencies (proximal and distal). If a sensory latency is reported instead of a velocity, the distance that was used (and whether that latency was measured to peak or onset) must be specified.

Since we are usually determining the sensory conduction velocity based on the latency, it is imperative to accurately measure the distance from the stimulator to the active electrode.

Table 21.1 EMG/NCS Reporting

Motor nerves
A. Latency
B. Amplitude
C. Conduction velocity
 	
Sensory nerves
A. Amplitude
B. Conduction velocity or distal latency
 	
Needle study
A. Insertional activity
  Increased (denervated muscle, myotonic discharges)
  Decreased (atrophy)
  Normal
B. Spontaneous activity
  Muscle generated
    Fibrillation potentials
    PSWs
    Myotonic discharges
    Complex repetitive discharges
  Neurally generated
  Fasciculations
    Myokymic discharges
    Cramps
    Neuromyotonic discharges
    Tremor
    Multiples
C. MUAP morphology
  Duration
  Polyphasicity
  Amplitude
D. Recruitment
  Increased firing frequency (decreased recruitment)
  Early
  Normal

EMG Findings

For EMG findings, report on insertional activity, activity at rest, MUAP (motor unit action potential) morphology and recruitment.

Insertional Activity

Increased insertional activity exists when there is a run of fibrillation potentials or positive sharp waves that only briefly persist beyond needle movement. (In order to be considered true fibrillation potentials or positive sharp waves, the waves should persist.) This is a somewhat subjective component and its accurate determination is dependent on the experience of the electromyographer. Myotonic discharges may also be noted on insertional activity. These are discharges that wax and wane in frequency and amplitude.

Spontaneous Activity

There are a variety of potentials that may be noted when the needle is at rest in the muscle. These potentials (and their significance) are described in Chapter 5.

SAMPLE REPORT

UNIVERSITY MEDICAL CENTER
Department of Physical Medicine and Rehabilitation
Anytown, N.Y.
(516) 123-4567

Patient:	Mary Smith	**Physician:**	A. Attending,
MR#:	1234567	**Resident:**	A. Resident
Ref Phys:	Dr. Jones	**Test date:**	8/20/04

DOB: 2/1/54
Sex: Female

Patient History:
This is a 48-year-old lady with a chief complaint of a morning pain in her right hand and tingling sensation in the right 1–3 digits for the last 2–3 months. Past medical history was significant for a whiplash injury about three years ago. She was seen at this hospital after the motor vehicle accident and discharged home on the same day. She doesn't take any medications except over-the-counter 'pain killers' and Lipitor for cholesterol control. The patient is right-handed. She works as a housekeeper. NCS/EMG was requested by her primary care physician to rule out right carpal tunnel syndrome.

Physical Examination:
Upon physical examination the patient appeared alert and oriented to person, place and time and was in no acute distress. There was no atrophy noted in bilateral thenar and hypothenar regions. There was full range of motion of both upper extremities. Motor exam of bilateral upper extremities revealed 5/5 strength to all upper extremity muscles except right grip was 4/5. There was a positive Tinel's sign elicited at the right wrist. Phalen's test was positive on the right. Upon cervical examination there was very mild paravertebral muscle spasm bilaterally. Spurling's test was negative bilaterally.

Figure 21.1 Sample Report

SAMPLE REPORT (*cont'd*)

ELECTRODIAGNOSTIC RESULTS:

Site	NR	Onset (ms)	Norm Onset (ms)	O-P Amp (mV)	Norm Amp (mV)	Segment Name	Dist (cm)	Vel (m/s)	Norm Vel (m/s)
Left Median (Abd Poll Brev)									
Wrist		3.36	<4.2	10.43	>4.0	Elbow-Wrist	18.5	52.56	>50.0
Elbow		6.88		11.00	>4.0				
Right Median (Abd Poll Brev)									
Wrist		4.61	<4.2	12.00	>4.0	Elbow-Wrist	16	46.51	>50.0
Elbow		8.05		12.34	>4.0				
Left Ulnar (Abd Dig Min)									
Wrist		2.81	<3.4	9.19	>4.0	B Elbow-Wrist	15	64.10	>50.0
B Elbow		5.16		6.02	>4.0	A Elbow-B Elbow	12	85.11	>50.0
A Elbow		6.56		9.89	>4.0				
Right Ulnar (Abd Dig Min)									
Wrist		3.13	<3.4	8.68	>4.0	B Elbow-Wrist	15.5	62.00	>50.0
B Elbow		5.63		10.11	>4.0	A Elbow-B Elbow	12	66.67	>50.0
A Elbow		7.42		9.80	>4.0				

Figure 21.1 (*cont'd*)

SAMPLE REPORT (cont'd)

Sensory Nerves

Site	NR	Onset (ms)	Norm Onset (ms)	O-P Amp (µV)	Norm Amp (µV)	Segment Name	Dist (cm)	Vel (m/s)	Norm Vel (m/s)	Comment
Left Median Sen D2 (2nd Digit)										
Mid Palm		0.91		50.21	>20.0	Mid Palm–2nd Digit	6	65.93	>45.0	
Wrist		2.28		38.20	>20.0	Wrist–2nd Digit	12	52.63	>44.0	
Right Median Sen D2 (2nd Digit)										
Mid Palm		0.88		43.01	>20.0	Mid Palm–2nd Digit	6	68.18	>45.0	
Wrist		3.09		18.34	>20.0	Wrist–2nd Digit	12	38.83	>44.0	
Left Ulnar Sen (5th Digit)										
Wrist		2.34		23.53	>18.0	Wrist–5th Digit	14.0	59.83		
Right Ulnar Sen (5th Digit)										
Wrist		2.47		24.52	>18.0	Wrist–5th Digit	14.0	56.68		

EMG

Side	Muscle	Nerve	Root	Ins Act	PSW	Fibs	Amp	Poly	Fascic	Recrt	Pt Coop	Comment
Right	Abd Poll Brev	Median	C8-T1	Nml	0	0	Nml	0	0	Nml	Nml	
Right	1st Dor Int	Ulnar	C8-T1	Nml	0	0	Nml	0	0	Nml	Nml	
Right	Cerv Para C6	Rami	C6	Nml	0	0	Nml	0	0	Nml	Nml	
Right	Cerv Para C7	Rami	C7	Nml	0	0	Nml	0	0	Nml	Nml	

Electrodiagnostic Evaluation:

Nerve conduction study of the motor and sensory divisions of bilateral median and ulnar nerves was done. Right median compound motor action potential (CMAP) showed increased distal latency with normal amplitude and conduction velocity. The left median and bilateral ulnar nerve CMAPs showed normal distal latency, amplitude and conduction velocity.

Figure 21.1 (cont'd)

SAMPLE REPORT *(cont'd)*

Right median sensory nerve action potential (SNAP) showed decreased amplitude and slowed conduction velocity across the wrist. The left median and bilateral ulnar SNAPs showed normal amplitude and conduction velocity.

Monopolar needle EMG of the right cervical paraspinal muscles and right abductor pollicis brevis and first dorsal interosseous muscles was performed. EMG of the muscles showed normal insertional activity with no spontaneous activity at rest, normal motor unit action potential morphology and normal recruitment pattern.

Impression:
This study showed electrodiagnostic evidence of right median nerve demyelinating neuropathy across the carpal tunnel involving both motor and sensory fibers. There are no signs of denervation in the right abductor pollicis brevis muscle. This is consistent with right mild-to-moderate carpal tunnel syndrome.

Thank you for the courtesy of this referral.

_____
A. Resident, MD
Resident Physician

I have performed this test with the resident and agree with the above interpretation and conclusion.

_____
A. Attending, M.D.
Attending Physician

Figure 21.1 *(cont'd)*

A **Figure 21.1**
(*cont'd*)

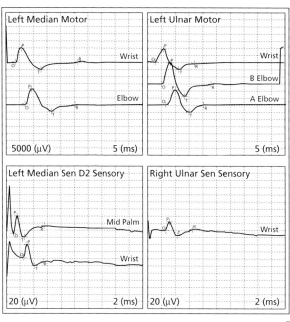

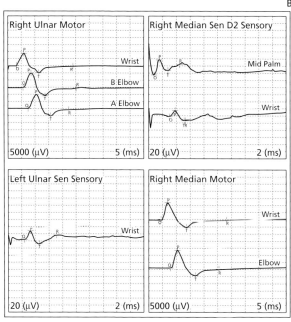

B

Motor Unit Action Potentials

Motor unit action potentials (MUAPs) should be classified as *normal* or *abnormal* based on *their morphology (appearance)*. If abnormal, the reason for the abnormality should be indicated. Abnormalities could include *duration, phases and/or amplitude*.

Motor Unit Recruitment

Recruitment abnormalities should be noted. For example, if there are few functioning motor units the remaining functioning units will fire at a higher frequency without other units being recruited. This abnormal (delayed) recruitment should be noted.

Table 21.1 summarizes the findings to be reported on in an NCS/EMG report.

Conclusion

Assuming you have completed a thorough electrodiagnostic examination, you want the pertinent information relayed to the referring physician. The conclusion should summarize your findings. Negative findings are sometimes also important. For example, a referring physician is requesting an EMG to rule out carpal tunnel syndrome. You find no evidence of carpal tunnel syndrome but you do find a C6 radiculopathy. It would be important to note that there is no electrodiagnostic evidence of carpal tunnel syndrome. (The term 'electrodiagnostic evidence' is important because although there may be *clinical* signs of nerve disorder, your conclusion should only report what the electrodiagnostic test reveals.)

Suggestions for possible treatments or interventions can be included in the report, but it is up to the referring physician to implement those suggestions. If further electro-diagnostic testing is indicated at a later time to help prognosticate, this should also be documented in the conclusion.

The sample report[1] (Fig. 21.1) is an example of how electrodiagnostic reports can be written.

REFERENCE

1.   Dumitru D. Electrodiagnostic Medicine. Philadelphia: Hanley & Belfus, 1995, p. 240.

22

Tables of Normals

Lyn Weiss, David Khanan, Chaim Shtock

It should be noted that each electrodiagnostic laboratory should develop its own standardized normal values. These tables should be used as a reference.

REFERENCES

1. Kimura J. Electrodiagnosis in Diseases of Nerve and Muscle, 2nd edn. New York: Oxford University Press, 1989.
2. Randall L, Braddom M. Physical Medicine and Rehabilitation. New York: WB Saunders, 1996.
3. DeLisa JA, Lee HJ, Baran EM, Lai K. Manual of Nerve Conduction Velocity and Clinical Neurophysiology, 3rd edn. New York: Raven Press, 1994.
4. Geiringer SR. Anatomic Localization for Needle Electromyography, 2nd edn. Philadelphia: Hanley & Belfus, 1999.
5. Tan JC. Practical Manual of Physical Medicine and Rehabilitation. New York: Mosby, 1998.
6. O'Young B. PM&R Secrets. Philadelphia: Hanley & Belfus, 1996.
7. DeLisa JA. Rehabilitation Medicine, 2nd edn. New York: Williams & Wilkins, 1988.
8. Dumitru D. Electrodiagnostic Medicine, 2nd edn. Philadelphia: Hanley & Belfus, 2002.

Table 22.1 Upper extremity – motor*

Nerve	Active electrode	Stimulation site	Distance (cm) from active to 1st stimulation site	Onset latency (ms)	Amplitude (mV)**	Segment name	Velocity m/s (meters/sec)
Median	Abductor pollicis brevis	Wrist Elbow	8	<4.2	>4.0 >4.0	Elbow-wrist	>50.0
Ulnar	Abductor digiti minimi	Wrist Below elbow (BE) Above elbow (AE)	8	<3.4	>4.0 >4.0 >4.0	BE-wrist AE-BE	>50.0 >50.0
Radial	Extensor indicis proprius	Forearm Erb's point	4	2.4 ± 0.5	14 ± 8.8	AE-EIP Erb's point-AE	61.6 ± 5.9 72 ± 6.3
Musculo-cutaneous	Distal to midpoint Biceps brachii	Erb's point	23.5–41.5	4.5 ± 0.6		Erb's point-Biceps brachii	
Axillary	Middle deltoid	Erb's point	14.8–26.5	3.9 ± 0.5		Erb's point-deltoid	

*Skin temperature should be maintained at 32°C.
**Side to side amplitude difference of >50% is significant, or >20% amplitude drop distal to proximal is significant.

Table 22.2 Upper extremity – sensory*

Nerve	Active electrode	Stimulation site	Distance (cm)	Onset latency (ms)	Amplitude µV (microvolts)	Segment name	Velocity (m/s)
Median	2nd digit	Mid palm Wrist	7 7	<1.9 <3.5	>20.0 >20.0	Mid palm–2nd digit Wrist–mid palm	>45.0 >45.0
Ulnar	5th digit	Wrist Below elbow Above elbow	14	<3.1	>18.0 >15.0 >14.0	Wrist–5th digit Below elbow–wrist Above elbow–below elbow	>44.0 >53.0 >54.0
Superficial radial	1st dorsal web space Forearm		14	1.8 ± 0.3 2.1 ± 0.3 2.4 ± 0.3	31 + 20 (13–60) 31 + 20 (13–60) 31 + 20 (13–60)	1st Web space–forearm	
Lateral antebrachial	Forearm	Elbow	12	1.8 ± 0.1 (1.6–2.1)	24.0 ± 7.2 (12–50)	Forearm–elbow	65 ± 3.6

*Skin temperature should be maintained at 32°C.

Table 22.3 Lower extremity – motor*

Nerve	Active electrode	Stimulation site	Distance (cm)	Onset latency (ms)	Amplitude (µV) (microvolts)	Segment name	Velocity (m/s)
Peroneal	Extensor digitorum brevis	Ankle					
		Fib head	?8	?<5.5	?>2.5	Fibular head–ankle	>40.0
		Popliteal				Popliteal–fibular head	>40.0
Post tibial	Abductor hallucis	Ankle	10	<6.0	>3.0	Knee–ankle	>40.0
		Knee					

*Skin temperature should be maintained at 30°C.

Table 22.4 Lower extremity – sensory*

Nerve	Active electrode	Stimulation site	Distance (cm)	Onset latency (ms)	Amplitude (µV) (microvolts)	Segment name	Velocity (m/s)
Sural	Lateral malleolus	Calf	14	<3.8	>10.0	Calf–lateral malleolus	>36.0
Lateral femoral cutaneous	1cm medial to anterior superior iliac spine (ASIS)	Anterior thigh	12–16	2.6 ± 0.2	10–25	ASIS–anterior thigh	47.9 ± 3.7
Superficial peroneal	Anterior to lateral malleolus	Anterolateral calf	14	3.4 ± 0.4	18.3 ± 8.0	Lateral malleolus to calf	51.2 ± 5.7

*Skin temperature should be maintained at 30°C.

Table 22.5 H-reflex* (see nomogram for normal values – Table 4.1)

Site	Active	Latency (ms)	Stimulation site
Medial gastrocnemius soleus muscle	Halfway from mid popliteal crease – proximal flare medial malleolus	28.0–35.0	Popliteal fossa (cathode proximal) use submaximal stimulation
*Skin temperature should be maintained at 30°C.			

Table 22.6 F-waves and F-ratio upper extremities

Motor nerve	Pick-up site	F-latency (ms)	F-ratio*
Median	Abductor pollicis brevis	Wrist 29.1 ± 2.3 Elbow 24.8 ± 2.0 Axilla 21.7 ± 2.8	0.7 < F < 1.3
Ulnar	Abductor digiti minimi	Wrist 30.5 ± 3.0 BE 26.0 ± 2.0 AE 23.5 ± 2.0 Axilla 11.2 ± 1.0	0.7 < F < 1.3
Peroneal	Extensor digitorum brevis	Ankle 51.3 ± 4.7 Knee 42.7 ± 4.0	0.7 < F < 1.3
Tibial	Abductor hallucis	Ankle 52.3 ± 4.3 Knee 43.5 ± 3.4	0.7 < F < 1.3

* F-ratio = $\dfrac{F - M - 1}{2M}$ (as measured at elbow or knee)

where F = F-wave latency, M = wave latency.

23

Reimbursement

Jay Weiss

This chapter is written to provide guidelines for electrodiagnostic reimbursement issues. It is difficult, in a few pages, to adequately cover all aspects of this topic. Two terms must be defined when discussing reimbursement – *coding* and *billing*. There are books and journals that deal exclusively with these issues. Coding is the process of transforming diagnoses and procedures into numeric codes, while billing is the process of transmitting the correct diagnosis and procedure codes to the payer. This chapter will cover the most commonly used electrodiagnostic procedures. Every effort has been made to use codes that are current as of the date of publication, however the codes used can and do change over time. Therefore, it is incumbent upon the physician to remain up to date on current acceptable coding and billing practices.

The electrodiagnostic evaluation is a complex, time-consuming examination requiring real-time interpretation of data and continual reassessment and modification of which nerves and muscles are to be tested. It also requires highly specialized computerized equipment, and complete familiarity with the technology. As such, it should be appropriately reimbursed for a test requiring this level of skill, training, knowledge, time and equipment.

The electrodiagnostic consultation is an extension of the neurologic portion of the physical examination. It is essential for the electromyographer to perform a history and physical examination as part of the study. If such an examination is performed and documented, it would be entirely appropriate to bill for the examination under the Medical Evaluation and Management Codes. These are the same codes used to describe office visits and consultations. Usually, Codes 99242–4 would be used.

Before we discuss billing we must tackle the issue of coding. Most insurance companies and Medicare carriers require all listed procedures and diagnoses to be provided in the form of numeric codes, because computers can more easily process these codes (rather than narrative descriptions). The importance of proper coding cannot be overstated. Insurance carriers will deny or reimburse electrodiagnostic procedures based on the diagnostic code used. Often there are several diagnosis codes that may fit a clinical picture. There are generalized codes for pain or numbness in a limb and more specific codes for peripheral entrapments or radiculopathies. In instances where there is neck pain and clinical evidence of radiculopathy, it is more important to use the radiculopathy code than the neck pain code because generic neck pain may or may not merit electrodiagnostic studies but radiculopathies most often will. There can be (and frequently is) more than one diagnostic code that is used.

Where Do These Codes Come From?

There are two books that are necessary for proper coding. For *diagnosis* codes, the book is called ICD-9 CM (International Classification of Diseases, 9th Edition[1]). ICD-9 codes generally do not change from year to year. The second book is the Current Procedural Terminology[2] (CPT) book that is published annually by the American Medical Association (AMA) and attempts to most accurately describe *procedures*. For the most commonly used electrodiagnostic codes, see Table 23.1. The AMA's CPT Manual frequently eliminates, revises and/or creates new codes. As a practical matter, some insurance carriers or systems may not recognize all current CPT codes; some may use eliminated codes. In specific instances it may be necessary to discuss individual coding questions with the carrier to find their closest acceptable code.

 Using the Procedure Codes

When billing for nerve studies it should be remembered that 95900 and 95904 are used for each nerve and therefore each code can be used more than once. Multiple stimulation sites on the same nerve are all part of one nerve study and should only be coded once. In other words, a median motor nerve study with electrodes over the abductor pollicis brevis and stimulations at the wrist, elbow, axilla and Erb's point counts as *one nerve study*. Median motor and sensory studies of both upper extremities and ulnar motor and sensory studies of both upper extremities would correctly be coded as 95900 four times and 95904 four times. If there were F-wave studies performed on both ulnar nerves (in addition to the median and ulnar motor and sensory nerves) then the proper billing would be:

95900 × 2 for the right and left median motor studies
95903 × 2 for the right and left ulnar motor nerve studies with F-waves
95904 × 4 for the right and left median and right and left ulnar sensory
        studies.

The 95860, 95861, 95863, 95864 codes include all muscles examined in an extremity along with related paraspinal areas. The CPT manual is not specific as to what constitutes an extremity however; if only one or two muscles are examined it is probably most appropriate to code this as 95870 – limited study of muscles in one extremity. Medicare requires that five muscles be examined to bill for an extremity.

Most carriers permit (and encourage) electronic submission. In these instances your diagnosis and procedure codes are the only information the carrier will receive from you. Some carriers may request additional documentation. In other instances the carrier may not realize that a Code (95900 – as an example) can be billed four times and they may only reimburse one study. A review of the explanation of benefits portion of the claim may show that a code was denied three times as 'repeat study' or 'previously billed'. In instances such as these it would be helpful to send your report along with a copy of the CPT page noting that the code is 'per nerve'. You may have to educate the carrier or the claims representative as to the definitions of codes.

While it is the physician's decision to determine his or her own fees for procedures, in many instances (including Medicare and managed care plans), a physician agrees to accept a predetermined fee schedule. In cases of Workers' Compensation and motor vehicle accidents most states have fixed fee schedules. The practitioner should be aware of the current testing fees in use in his or her geographic area.

Table 23.1 Current procedural terminology (CPT™) codes in electrodiagnostic medicine[2]

95860	Needle electromyography, one extremity with or without related paraspinal areas
95861	Needle electromyography, two extremities with or without related paraspinal areas
95863	Needle electromyography, three extremities with or without related paraspinal areas
95864	Needle electromyography, four extremities with or without related paraspinal areas
95867	Needle electromyography, cranial nerve supplied muscles, unilateral
95868	Needle electromyography, cranial nerve supplied muscles, bilateral
95869	Needle electromyography; thoracic paraspinal muscles
95870	Limited study of muscles in one extremity or non-limb (axial) muscles (unilateral or bilateral), other than thoracic paraspinal, cranial nerve supplied muscles, or sphincters
Nerve conduction studies	
95900	Nerve conduction, amplitude and latency/velocity study, each nerve; motor, without F-wave study
95903	Nerve conduction, amplitude and latency/velocity study, each nerve; motor with F-wave study
95904	Nerve conduction, amplitude and latency/velocity study, each nerve; motor with F-wave study, each nerve; sensory
95934	H-reflex, amplitude and latency study; record gastrocnemius/soleus muscle
95936	Record muscle other than gastrocnemius/soleus muscle

 ## Who Can Perform Testing?

The details of electrodiagnostic studies are discussed elsewhere in this text. In terms of reimbursement, it is important to note that a needle EMG test is a dynamic test that is individualized to the clinical circumstance. The EMG portion of the test must be performed by a physician, as opposed to a technician, and is interpreted in real-time as it is being performed. During the study, different muscles may or may not be examined depending on the results of the study to that point. The working diagnosis is continually modified and re-examined based on the findings. Therefore the examination may be altered to confirm or refute different diagnoses.

As opposed to needle EMG, a technician, with physician supervision, can perform nerve conduction studies. It is important however, to note that it is the physician who must dictate the design of the study (choice of nerves) to fit the clinical circumstances and is ultimately responsible for the analysis of the study. A physician should be available to confirm or refute any abnormal or unexpected electromyographic findings. Both the electromyographer and the technician should be aware of the numerous technical factors that can give false results.

In general, the EMG data cannot be recorded in order to be independently reviewed and separately interpreted as can, for instance, an MRI of the spine. In this way it is different from many other diagnostic tests. It is most similar to a physical examination where the only recording of the data is by the physician's independent record of the encounter. Thus, it can be seen that the validity of any electrodiagnostic study is totally dependent on the knowledge, experience and integrity of the electromyographer reporting the data.

Overuse of Studies

An electrodiagnostic consultation can be an expensive battery of tests and unfortunately there have been problems with overuse and inappropriate use of electrodiagnostic studies. The cost of these studies, along with instances of inappropriate use and overuse, make these studies likely to come under close scrutiny. Ultimately, this can lead to insurance denials or partial denials of payment for appropriate studies. Thus, it is important to be sure that the electrodiagnostic study fits the clinical picture.

An 'adequate' number of nerve studies and needle insertions insure the greatest degree of accuracy without undue discomfort or inappropriate expense. EMG testing of the extremity should be sufficient to refute or confirm a diagnosis. In most instances EMG should include the most symptomatic muscle or muscles (generally the weakest). If a symptomatic extremity is normal on EMG, examination of the asymptomatic extremity is not likely to be needed.

Nerve studies should be performed to provide specific information. Generally one or two motor and sensory nerves are adequate in ruling out a generalized peripheral neuropathy. Beyond that, specific nerves can be helpful in evaluating a peripheral entrapment versus a more proximal lesion. In instances where a diagnosis of root avulsion is being considered, sensory nerve studies can be crucial. In all cases there should be reasons based on the clinical circumstances for the nerve studies performed (Table 23.2).

 Peer Review Process

If there are questions as to the appropriateness of electrodiagnostic studies, the American Board of Electrodiagnostic Medicine (ABEM) recommends the use of a peer review process. A physician with training in electrodiagnostic medicine should perform the peer review process for electrodiagnostic studies. Such a physician is almost always either a neurologist or a physiatrist. It is most appropriate for this specialist to be a practicing electromyographer who would therefore utilize the same criteria employed in his or her clinical practice. The ABEM has guidelines which suggest the number of nerve studies that should be adequate in greater than 90% of studies for a particular diagnosis. Studies that exceed these numbers could trigger peer review or other scrutiny (see Table 23.3).

While the actual electrodiagnostic study cannot be reviewed for purposes of confirming or refuting the findings, a review of electrodiagnostic reports can, in some circumstances, be helpful. A review can address whether there were indications for the testing and it can also note instances where the study was poorly designed. This can include a study that was too limited to fit the clinical circumstances or inadequate in its muscle selection. A review can address whether the conclusions were or were not supported by the data.

 Summary

It is not enough merely to be a good electromyographer. The appropriate diagnoses and procedure codes are necessary for obtaining proper reimbursement. The procedures performed should fit the clinical circumstances and should be adequate without being excessive. The procedures and indications should be adequately documented. By satisfying these criteria, the likelihood of proper reimbursement is maximized.

Table 23.2 AAEM recommended policy for electrodiagnostic medicine[3]; diagnosis/unit usage table of the recommended policy (see Table 23.1)

Indication	Needle electromyography CPT™ 95860-95864 and 95867-95870 Number of services (tests)	Nerve conduction studies CPT™ 95900, 95903, 95904 Motor NCS with and/or without F-wave	Sensory NCS	Other electromyographic studies CPT™ 95934, 95937, 95936 H-reflex	Neuromuscular junction testing (repetitive stimulation)
Carpal tunnel (unilateral)	1	3	4		
Carpal tunnel (bilateral)	2	4	6		
Radiculopathy	2	3	2	2	
Mononeuropathy	1	3	3	2	
Polyneuropathy/ mononeuropathy multiplex	3	4	4	2	
Myopathy	2	2	2		2
Motor neuronopathy (e.g., ALS)	4	4	2		2
Plexopathy	2	4	6	2	
Neuromuscular junction	2	2	2		3
Tarsal tunnel syndrome (unilateral)	1	4	4		
Tarsal tunnel syndrome (bilateral)	2	5	6		
Weakness, fatigue, cramps, or twitching (focal)	2	3	4		2
Weakness, fatigue, cramps, or twitching (general)	4	4	4		2
Pain, numbness, or tingling (unilateral)	1	3	4	2	
Pain, numbness, or tingling (bilateral)	2	4	6	2	

Used with permission © 2002 AAEM

REFERENCES

1. International Classification of Diseases, 9th Revision, Clinical Modification. Physician ICD-9-CM.2002. AMA Press Chicago; 2001, Ingenix, Inc.
2. Current Procedural Terminology, CPT 2003. AMA Press, Chicago.
3. AAEM Recommended Policy for Electrodiagnostic Medicine, Revised 2002. www.aaem.net/position_statements.htm.

Glossary of EMG Terms

Action potential
an electrical potential that moves along an axon or muscle fiber membrane.

Action potential morphology
the electrical representation of the nerve stimulation – seen as a small hill on the screen – commonly called a waveform.

Amplitude
the maximal height of the action potential (can be measured baseline to peak or peak to trough); expressed in millivolts (mV) or microvolts (μV).

Antidromic
when the electrical impulse travels in the opposite direction of normal physiologic conduction (e.g., conduction of a motor nerve electrical impulse away from the muscle and toward the spine).

Axonotmesis
injury to the axon of a nerve but not the supporting connective tissue. Results in Wallerian degeneration distal to the injury.

Compound motor action potential (CMAP)
summation of action potentials recorded over a muscle following stimulation of a motor nerve.

Conduction block
failure of an action potential to propagate past an area of injury, generally due to focal demyelination.

Conduction velocity
a measure of how fast the fastest part of the impulse travels (can also be referred to as a motor conduction velocity or a sensory conduction velocity).

Electrodiagnostic studies
includes many tests, e.g., nerve conduction studies (NCS) and electromyography (EMG) – is a physiological assessment of the electrical functioning of nerves and/or muscles.

F-wave
a compound muscle action potential evoked from antidromically stimulated motor nerve fibers using a supramaximal electrical stimulus. Generally represents only a small percentage of fibers and therefore much smaller than M-wave.

Fasciculation potential
spontaneous electrical potential originating in the nerve and which can have the morphology of a motor unit action potential.

Fibrillation potential
spontaneous potential found on EMG at rest; biphasic, initially positive deflection, originating in the muscle.

Frequency
cycles per second (frequently abbreviated Hertz or Hz).

H-reflex
a compound muscle action potential evoked through orthodromic stimulation of sensory fibers and orthodromic activation of motor fibers. This is evoked with a submaximal stimulation and disappears with supramaximal stimulation. It is found in normal adults only in the gastrocnemius-soleus and flexor carpi radialis muscles. The response is thought to be due to a mono- or oligosynaptic spinal reflex (Hoffmann reflex).

Insertional activity
the electrical activity generated as a result of disruption of the muscle membrane by a needle.

Late response
an evoked potential with a latency longer than an M-wave; includes H-reflexes and F-waves.

Latency
time interval between the onset of a stimulus and the onset of a response.

M-wave
muscle action potential evoked by stimulating a motor nerve.

Miniature endplate potential
potential produced spontaneously by the release of one quanta of acetylcholine from the presynaptic axon terminal.

Motor point
where the nerve enters the muscle (endplate zone).

Motor unit
includes the anterior horn cell, its axon, neuromuscular junction and all the muscle fibers innervated by that axon.

Myokymic discharge
motor unit action potentials that fire repetitively (often referred to as sounding like marching soldiers).

Myopathic recruitment
increased number and early recruitment of motor unit action potentials for the strength of contraction; motor units are generally of small amplitude. Frequently seen in myopathies.

Myotonic discharge
high frequency discharges whose amplitude and frequency wax and wane (sometimes referred to as 'dive bombers').

Nerve conduction studies (NCS)
assessment of functioning of nerves via electrical stimulation.

Neurapraxia
a lesion where conduction block is present. The axon remains intact.

Neurotmesis
a *complete* injury of a nerve (such as a transection) involving the myelin, axon and all the supporting structures.

Orthodromic
when the electrical impulse travels in the same direction as normal physiologic conduction (e.g., when a motor nerve electrical impulse is transmitted toward the muscle and away from the spine).

Positive sharp wave
primarily monophasic spontaneous potential found on EMG at rest, initially positive deflection with a characteristic 'V' formation.

Recruitment
the orderly addition of motor units with increasing voluntary muscle contraction.

Sensory nerve action potential (SNAP)
summation of action potentials recorded from the nerve following stimulation of a sensory nerve.

Stimulus
an electrical depolarization of a nerve initiating an action potential. A stimulus can be supramaximal or submaximal.

Submaximal stimulus
an electrical stimulus that results in the initiation of an action potential in some (but not all) of the nerve fibers. Increasing the intensity of a submaximal stimulus will change the appearance of the CMAP or SNAP.

Supramaximal stimulus
an electrical stimulus that results in the initiation of an action potential in all of the fibers of the targeted nerve. Increasing the

intensity of a supramaximal stimulus will not change the appearance of the CMAP or SNAP (but may shorten the latency).

Temporal dispersion
long duration, low amplitude potential due to extreme variations in the conduction velocities of individual nerve fibers contributing to the action potential.

Appendix 1

Figures for Table 4.3 Nerve conduction studies setup

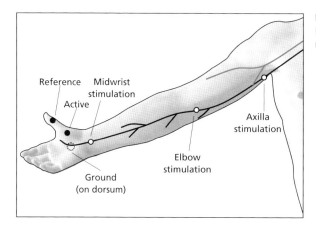

Figure A1.1
Median nerve – motor.

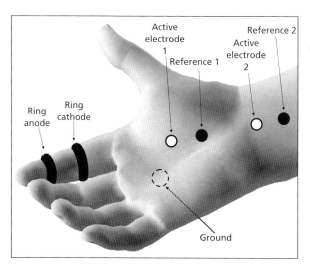

Figure A1.2
Median nerve – sensory (orthodromic).

Figure A1.3
Median nerve –
sensory
(antidromic).

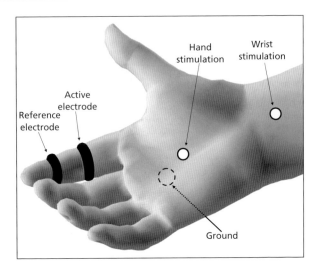

Figure A1.4 Ulnar
nerve – motor.

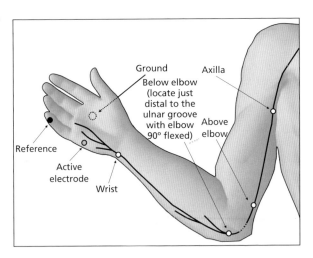

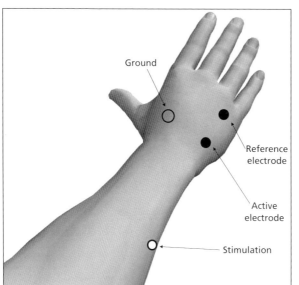

Figure A1.5 Dorsal ulnar cutaneous nerve – sensory (orthodromic).

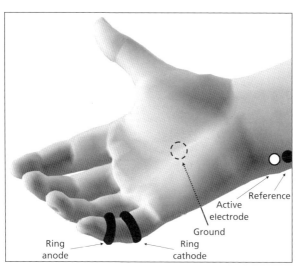

Figure A1.6 Ulnar nerve – sensory (orthodromic).

Figure A1.7 Ulnar
nerve – sensory
(antidromic).

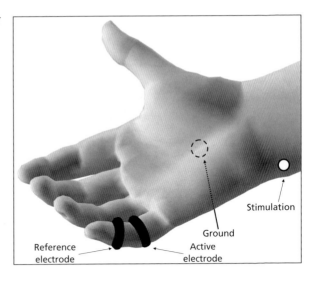

Figure A1.8
Radial nerve –
sensory
(antidromic).

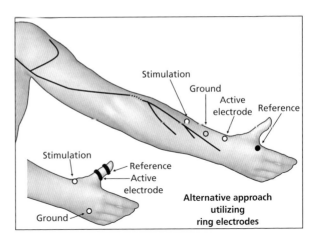

Figure A1.9
Radial nerve –
motor.

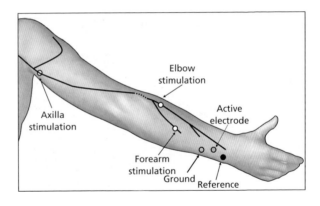

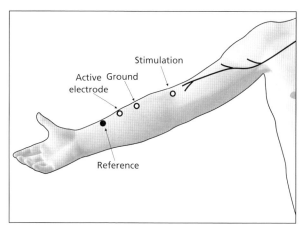

Figure A1.10
Musculocutaneous nerve – sensory (antidromic) (lateral antebrachial cutaneous nerve).

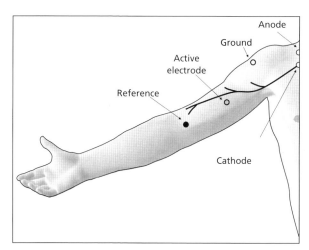

Figure A1.11
Musculocutaneous nerve – motor.

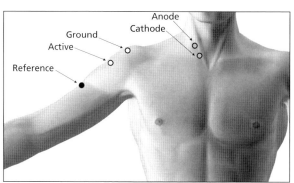

Figure A1.12
Axillary nerve – motor.

Figure A1.13
Peroneal nerve –
motor.

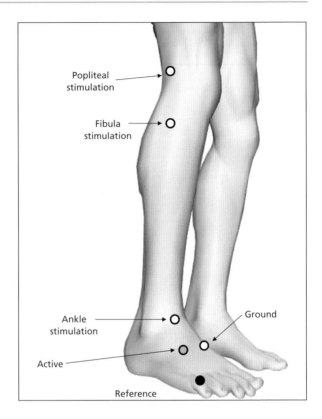

Popliteal
stimulation

Fibula
stimulation

Ankle
stimulation

Ground

Active

Reference

Figure A1.14
Sural nerve –
sensory.

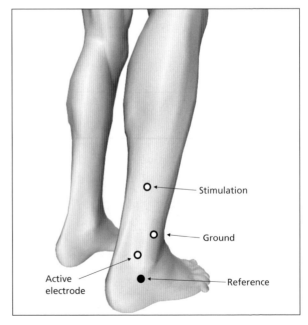

Stimulation

Ground

Active
electrode

Reference

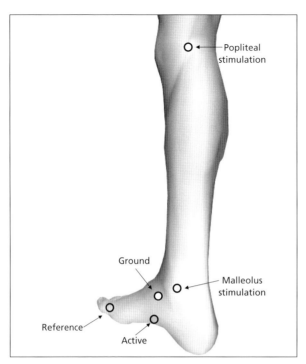

Figure A1.15
Tibial nerve –
motor to
abductor hallucis.

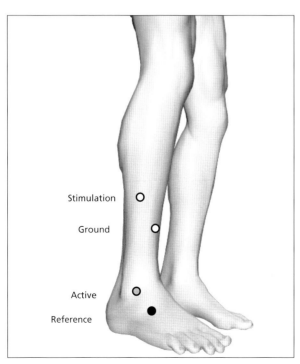

Figure A1.16
Superficial
peroneal nerve –
sensory
(antidromic).

Figure A1.19
Sciatic nerve –
motor.

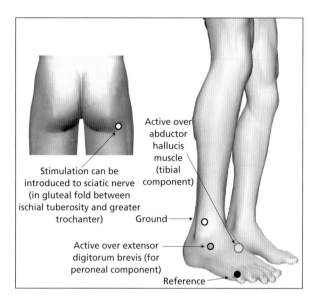

Active over
abductor
hallucis
muscle
(tibial
component)

Stimulation can be
introduced to sciatic nerve
(in gluteal fold between
ischial tuberosity and greater
trochanter)

Ground

Active over extensor
digitorum brevis (for
peroneal component)

Reference

Figure A1.20
Lateral femoral
cutaneous nerve –
sensory
(antidromic).

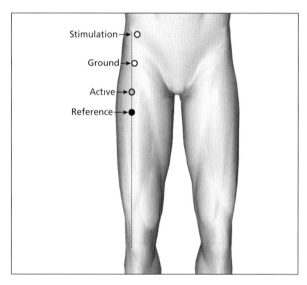

Stimulation

Ground

Active

Reference

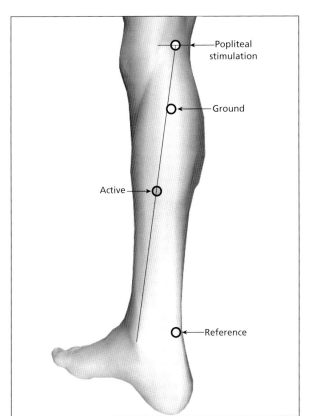

Figure A1.19
H-reflex.

Appendix 2

Figures to Table 5.4 Common muscles – innervation, location and needle placement

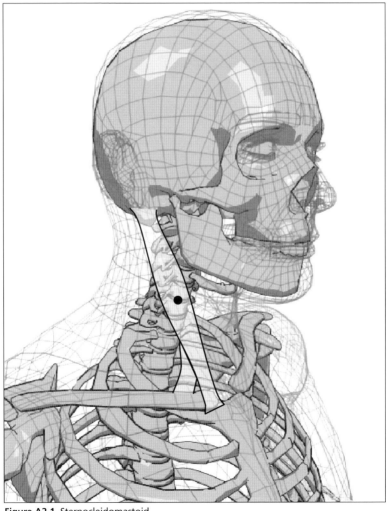

Figure A2.1 Sternocleidomastoid.

Figure A2.2
Trapezius.

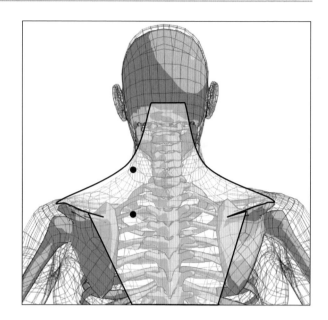

Figure A2.3
Rhomboid major
(RMa), rhomboid
minor (RMi).

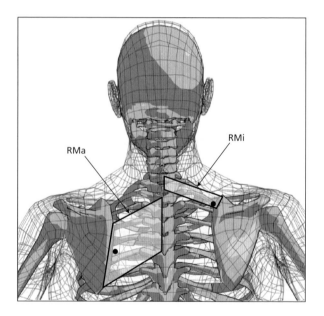

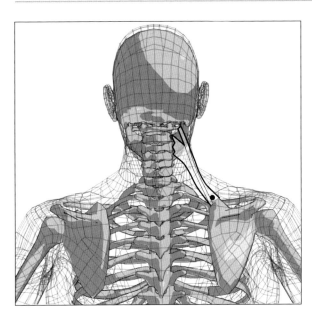

Figure A2.4
Levator scapula.

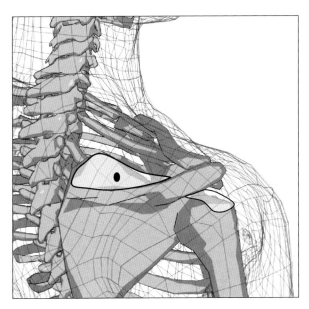

Figure A2.5
Supraspinatus.

Figure A2.6
Infraspinatus.

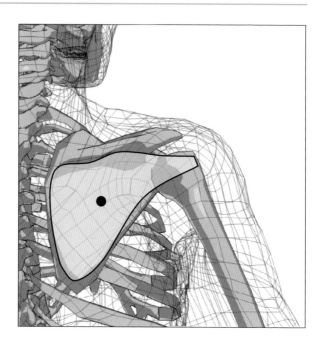

Figure A2.7 Teres major.

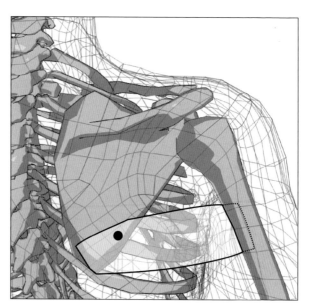

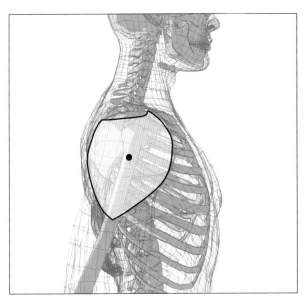

Figure A2.8
Deltoid.

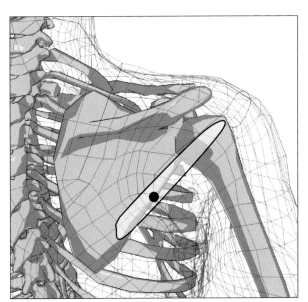

Figure A2.9 Teres minor.

Figure A2.10
Coracobrachialis.

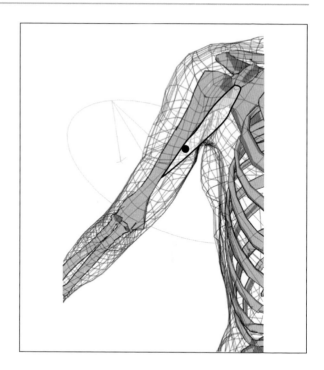

Figure A2.11
Biceps brachii.

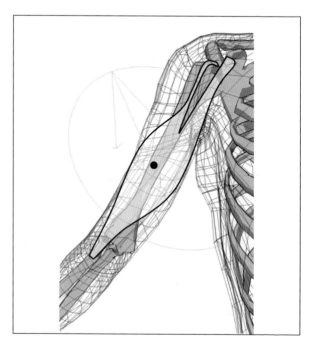

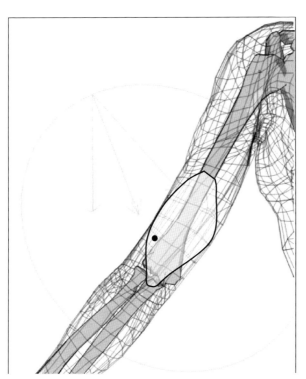

Figure A2.12
Brachialis.

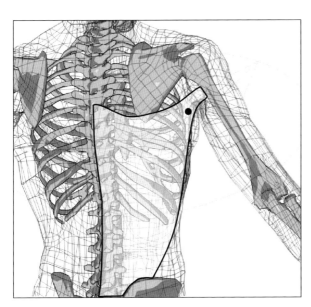

Figure A2.13
Latissimus dorsi.

Figure A2.14
Serratus anterior.

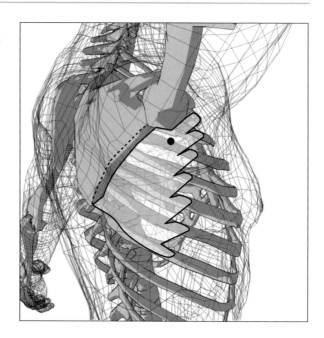

Figure A2.15
Triceps.

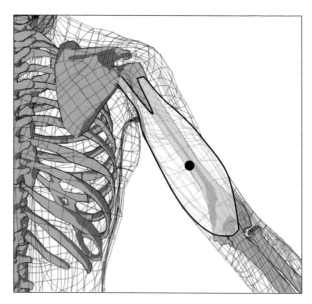

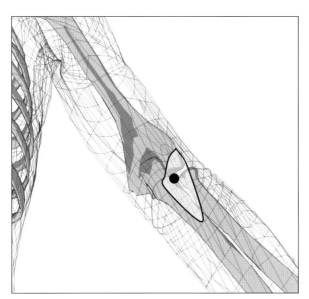

Figure A2.16
Anconeus.

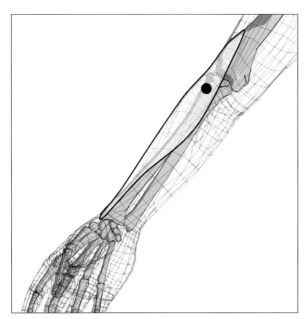

Figure A2.17
Brachioradialis.

Figure A2.18
Extensor carpi
radialis.

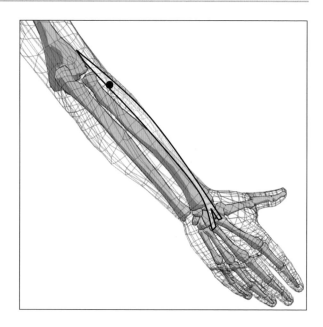

Figure A2.19
Supinator.

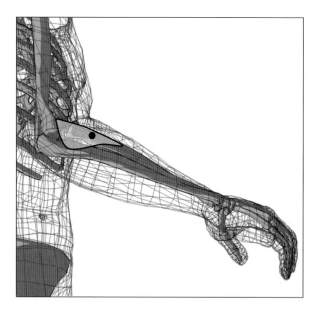

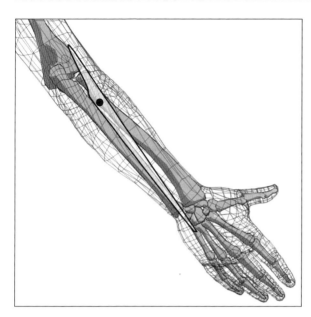

Figure A2.20
Extensor carpi
ulnaris.

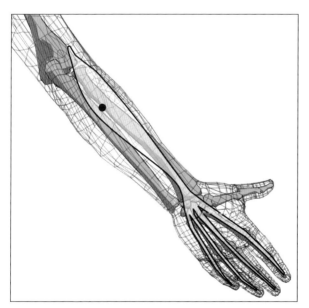

Figure A2.21
Extensor
digitorum.

Figure A2.22
Extensor
digitorum minimi.

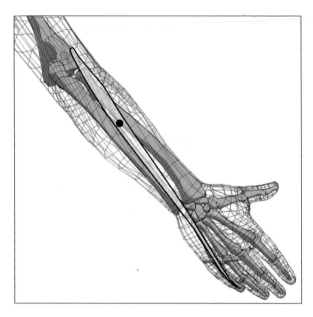

Figure A2.23
Abductor pollicis
longus.

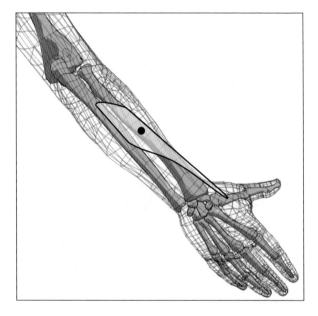

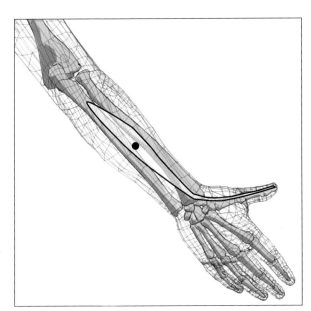

Figure A2.24
Extensor pollicis longus.

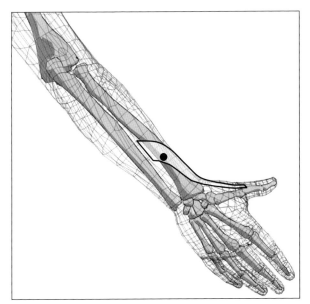

Figure A2.25
Extensor pollicis brevis.

Figure A2.26
Extensor indicis.

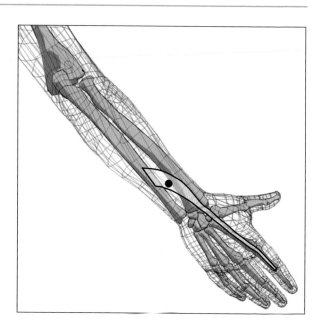

Figure A2.27
Pronator teres
(PT), pronator
quadratus (PQ).

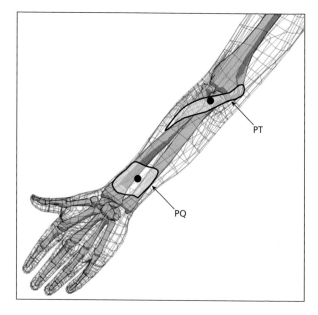

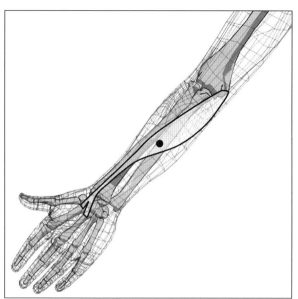

Figure A2.28
Flexor carpi radialis.

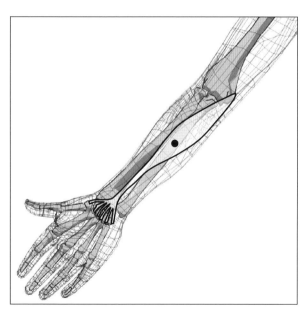

Figure A2.29
Palmaris longus.

Figure A2.30
Flexor digitorum
superficialis.

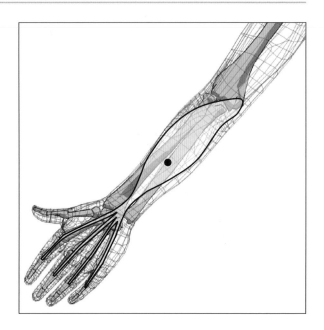

Figure A2.31
Flexor digitorum
profundus.

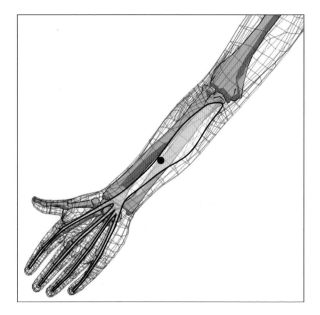

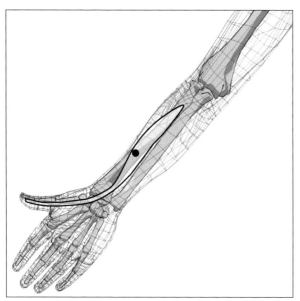

Figure A2.32
Flexor pollicis longus.

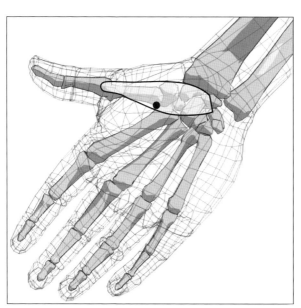

Figure A2.33
Abductor pollicis brevis.

Figure A2.34
Opponens pollicis.

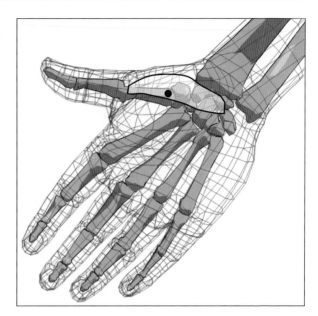

Figure A2.35
Flexor pollicis brevis.

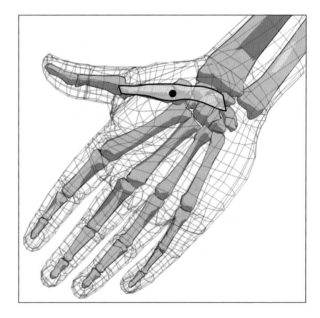

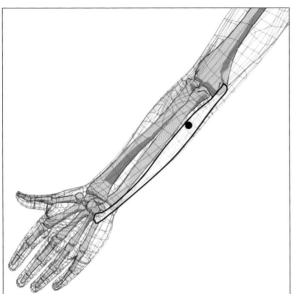

Figure A2.36
Flexor carpi ulnaris.

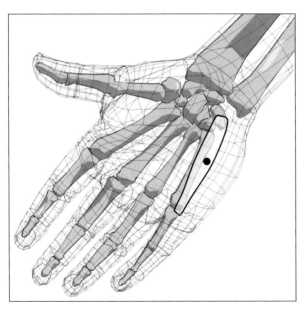

Figure A2.37
Abductor digiti minimi.

Figure A2.38
Opponens digiti
minimi.

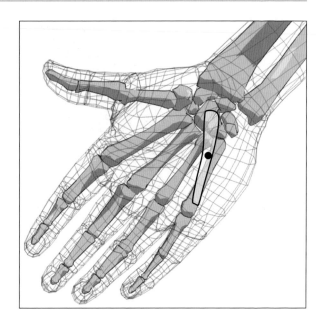

Figure A2.39
Flexor digiti
minimi.

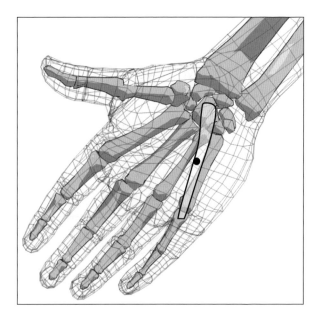

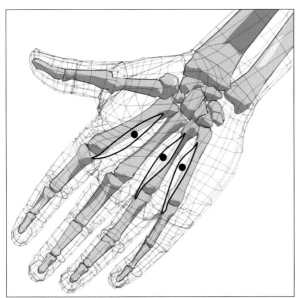

Figure A2.40
Palmar interossei.

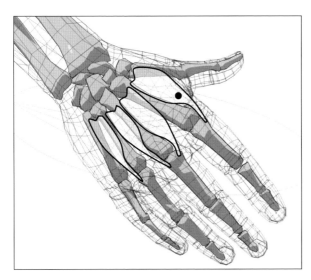

Figure A2.41
Dorsal interossei.

Figure A2.42
Adductor pollicis.

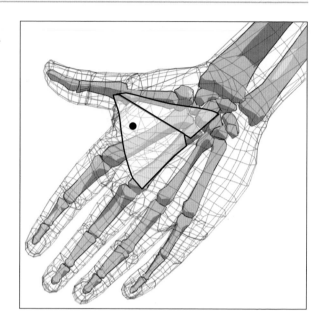

Figure A2.43
Lumbricals.

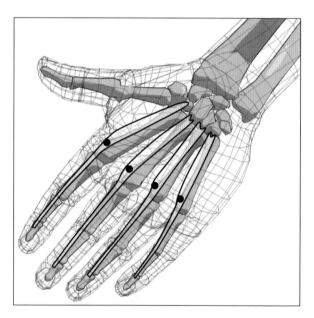

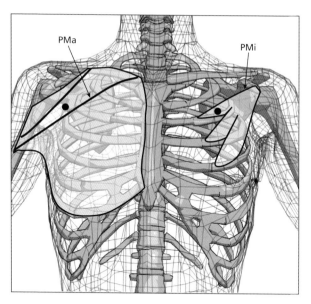

Figure A2.44
Pectoralis major
(PMa), pectoralis
minor (PMi).

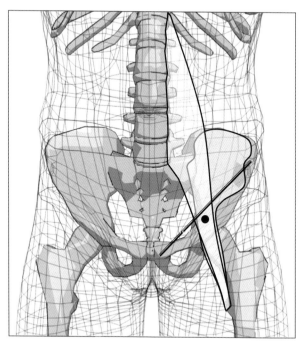

Figure A2.45
Iliopsoas.

Figure A2.46
Muscles of the anterior thigh.

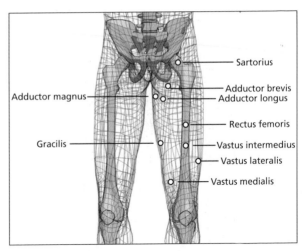

Sartorius

Adductor brevis
Adductor longus

Adductor magnus

Rectus femoris

Gracilis

Vastus intermedius

Vastus lateralis

Vastus medialis

Figure A2.47
Sartorius.

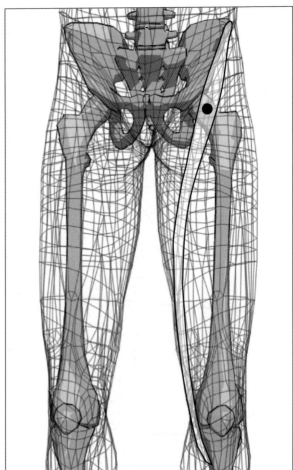

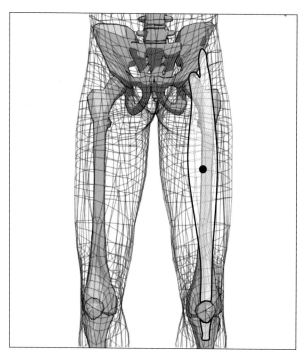

Figure A2.48
Rectus femoris.

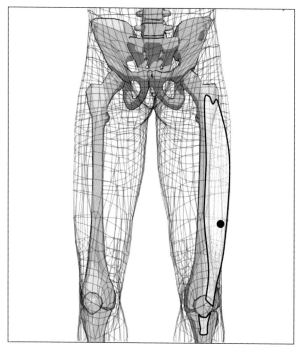

Figure A2.49
Vastus lateralis.

Figure A2.50
Vastus
intermedius.

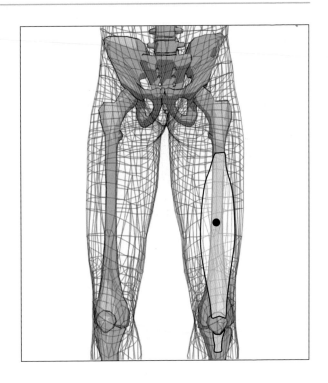

Figure A2.51
Vastus medialis.

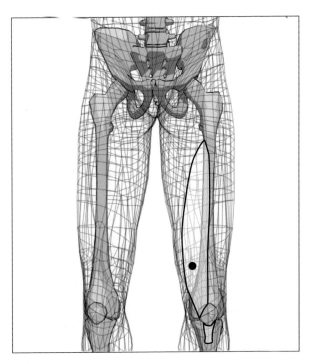

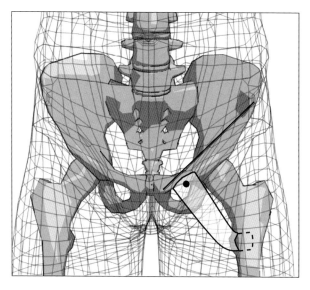

Figure A2.52
Pectineus.

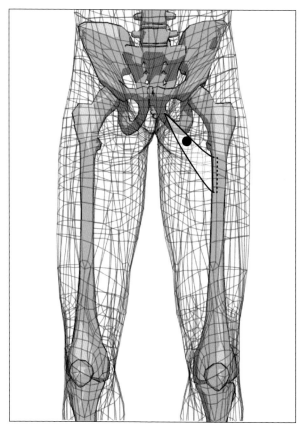

Figure A2.53
Adductor brevis.

Figure A2.54
Adductor longus.

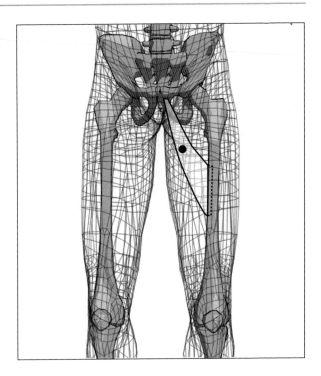

Figure A2.55
Gracilis.

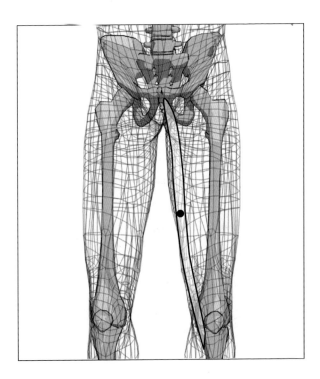

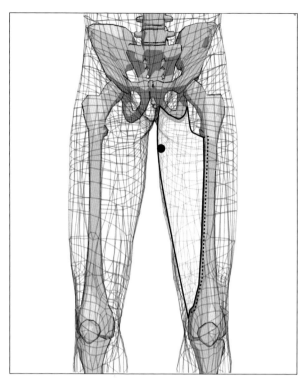

Figure A2.56
Adductor
magnus.

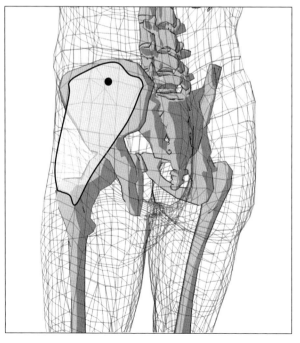

Figure A2.57
Gluteus medius.

Figure A2.58
Gluteus minimus.

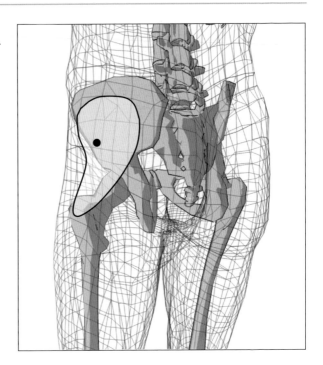

Figure A2.59
Tensor fascia latae.

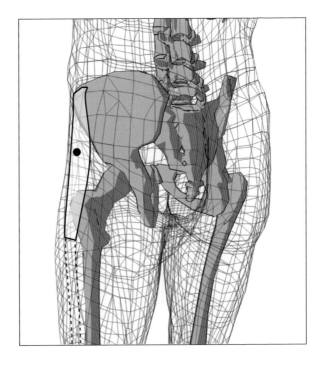

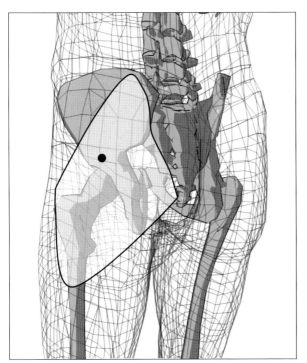

Figure A2.60
Gluteus maximus.

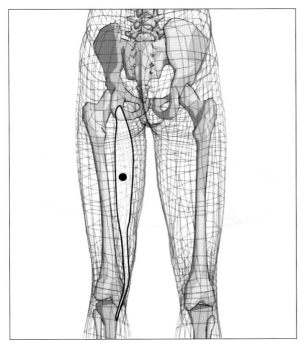

Figure A2.61
Semitendinosus.

Figure A2.62
Semimembranosus.

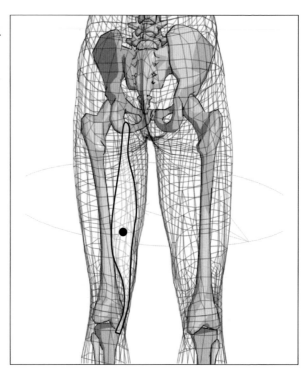

Figure A2.63
Biceps femoris.

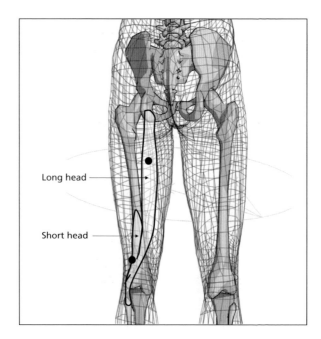

Long head

Short head

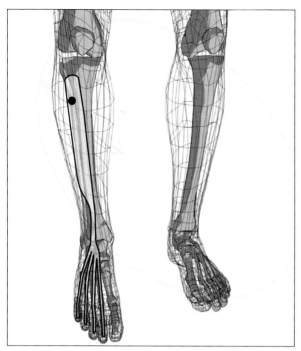

Figure A2.64
Extensor
digitorum longus.

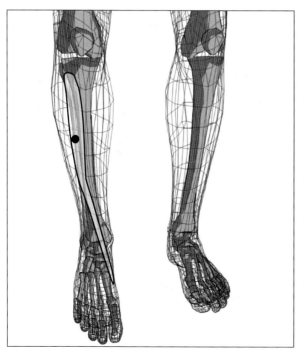

Figure A2.65
Tibialis anterior.

Figure A2.66
Extensor hallucis
longus.

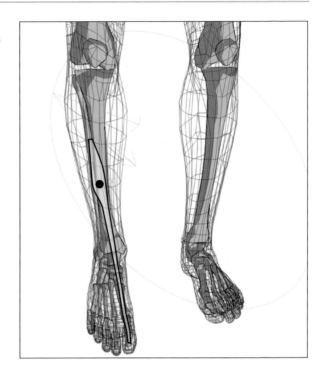

Figure A2.67
Peroneus tertius.

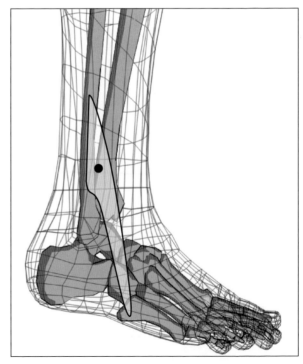

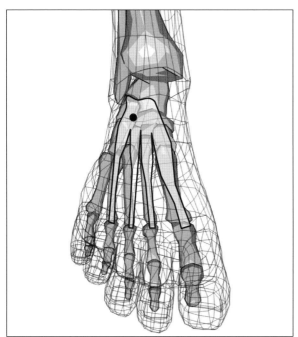

Figure A2.68
Extensor
digitorum brevis.

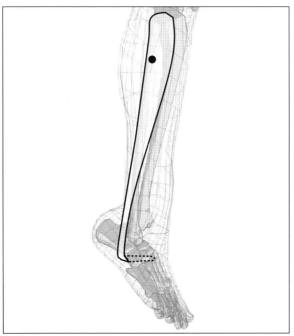

Figure A2.69
Peroneus longus.

Figure A2.70
Peroneus brevis.

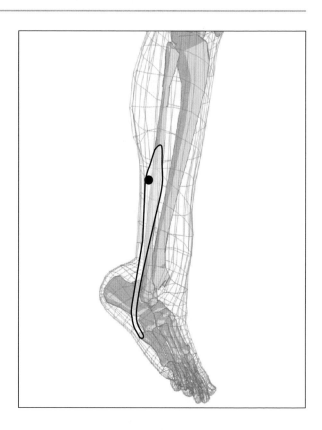

Figure A2.71
Medial lateral
gastrocnemius.

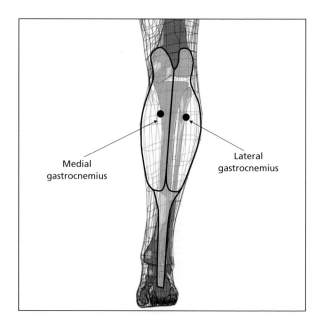

Medial
gastrocnemius

Lateral
gastrocnemius

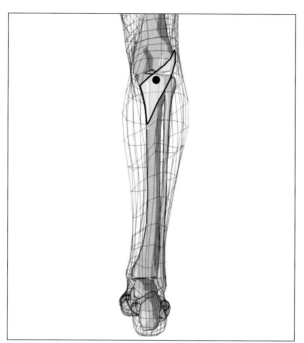

Figure A2.72
Popliteus.

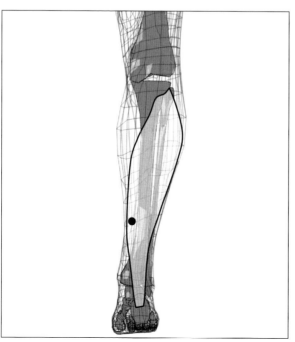

Figure A2.73
Soleus.

Figure A2.74
Muscles of the calf.

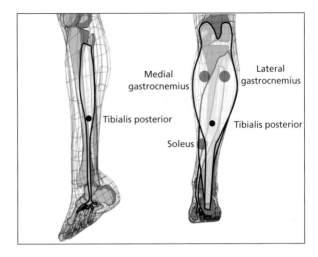

Medial gastrocnemius

Lateral gastrocnemius

Tibialis posterior

Tibialis posterior

Soleus

Figure A2.75
Flexor hallucis longus.

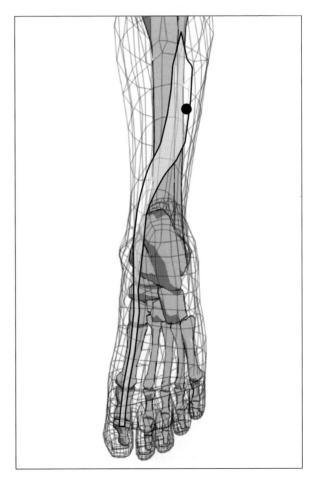

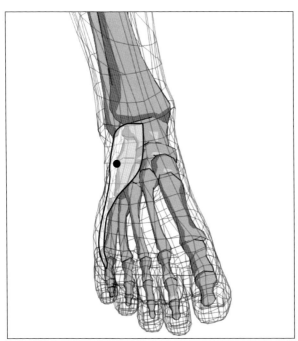

Figure A2.76
Abductor digiti minimi.

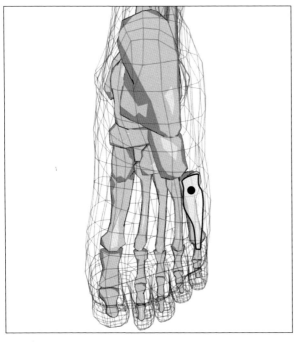

Figure A2.77
Flexor digiti minimi (plantar surface).

Figure A2.78
Dorsal interossei.

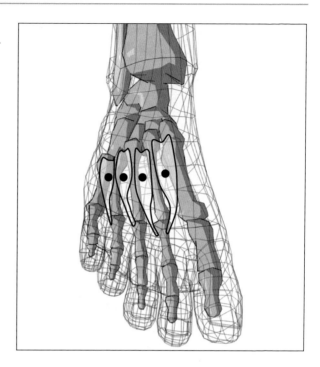

Figure A2.79
Plantar interossei
(plantar surface).

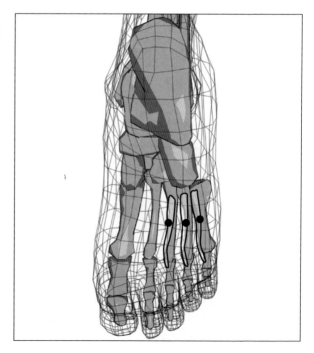

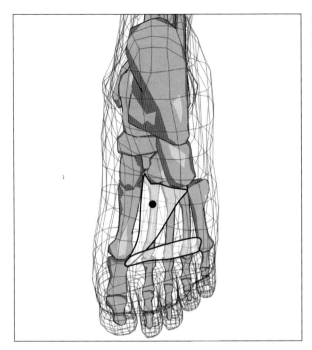

Figure A2.80
Adductor hallucis
(plantar surface).

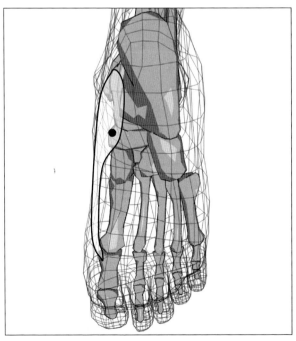

Figure A2.81
Abductor hallucis
(plantar surface).

Figure A2.82
Flexor digitorum
brevis (plantar
surface).

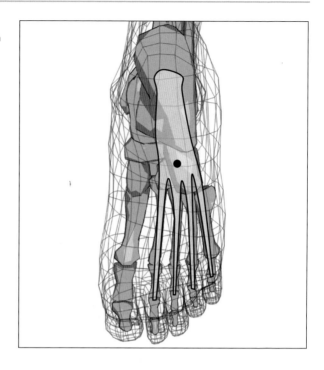

Figure A2.83
Flexor hallucis
brevis (plantar
surface).

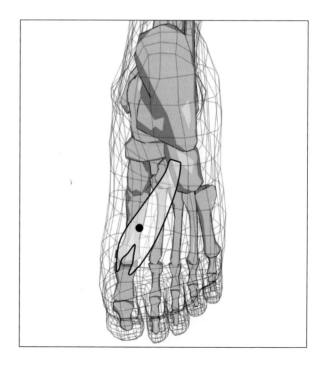

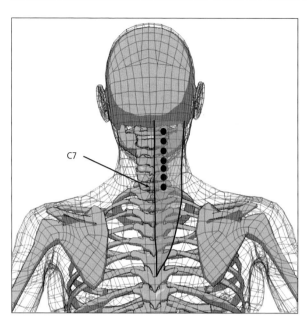

Figure A2.84
Cervical paraspinal.

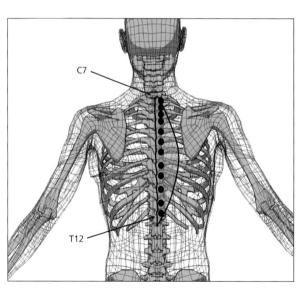

Figure A2.85
Thoracic paraspinal.

Figure A2.86
Lumbosacral
paraspinal.

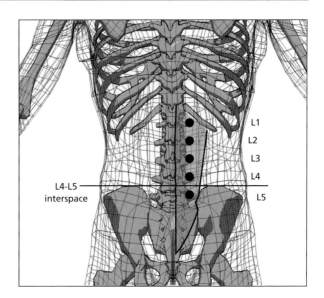

Index

267